Rosemary Gladstar's

Herbal Remedies *for* MEN'S HEALTH

The mission of Storey Communications is to serve our customers by publishing practical information that encourages personal independence in harmony with the environment.

This publication is intended to provide educational information for the reader on the covered subject. It is not intended to take the place of personalized medical counseling, diagnosis, and treatment from a trained health professional.

Edited by Deborah Balmuth and Robin Catalano
Cover design by Carol Jessop, Black Trout Design, and Meredith Maker
Back cover photograph by A. Blake Gardner
Cover and interior illustrations by Laura Tedeschi
Text design by Carol Jessop, Black Trout Design
Text production by Susan B. Bernier
Indexed by Nan Badgett, Word•a•bil•i•ty

Printed in Canada by Webcom Limited
10 9 8 7 6 5 4 3 2

Library of Congress Cataloging-in-Publication Data

Gladstar, Rosemary.
    [Herbal remedies for men's health]
    Rosemary Gladstar's Herbal remedies for men's health.
        p.   cm.
    Includes bibliographical references and index.
    ISBN 1-58017-151-6 (pbk. : alk. paper)
    1. Men — Health and hygiene.   2. Herbs — Therapeutic use.   3. Men —
Diseases—Alternative treament.   I. Title.
    RA777.8.G595   1999
    615'.321'081—dc21   99-19956
                                                                              CIP

Dedication

To my dad, Robert Karr, the sweetest, most gentle man I've ever known, my son, Jason Elan Colvard, for sharing the adventure, and my Dirt Man . . . Deeply honored you each are in this wild woman's heart.

Acknowledgments

This book would not have been possible without the input of the caring circle of men in my life. They not only offered their opinions and suggestions, but volunteered their willing hands through this period of intense writing. Wood got stacked. Snow was plowed. Meals were cooked, and animals were cared for. And even my house was cleaned. Nice guys!

Thanks especially to: Robert Chartier, Sage Mountain Earth Steward and Land Manager; Karl Slick; Matthais Reisen; David Bryant; and Jason Colvard. To those men in the herbal community who are offering classes on men's health, I applaud your pioneering efforts. Thanks to these teachers: Ryan Drum, James Green, David Winston, and Christopher Hobbs.

CONTENTS

Chapter One 1
New Perspectives on Men's Health

Chapter Two 7
Commonsense Guidelines for Good Health

Chapter Three 13
Making and Using Herbal Remedies

Chapter Four 25
The Man's Herbal Medicine Chest

Chapter Five 51
Formulas Especially for Men

Chapter Six 63
Remedies for Specific Ailments

Recommended Reading 85

Resources 86

United Plant Savers At-Risk List 89

Index 90

New Perspectives on Men's Health

The book section in my library labeled "Women's Health" is getting rather crowded and books are beginning to topple each other. Not surprisingly, there's been a plethora of books published on women's herbs, health, and healing in the past few years. Written by caring practitioners, both men and women, many of the topics are excellent. They focus their attention on women's health issues and offer the reader a rich tapestry of views and information.

Unfortunately, the same cannot be said for information on men's health. There are few published articles, fewer books, and very little information circulating. My book section on men's health is dismally empty except for one brave classic, *The Male Herbal: Health Care for Men and Boys* by James Green. Published in 1991, this book was groundbreaking not only because it was the first book of its kind on the subject, but also because it presented Green's revolutionary and rather unique views on male health.

So why isn't there more information available? Different approaches, different views to draw upon? Aren't men interested? Don't they get sick? They will tell you they don't, but when one looks at the statistics of male health in the United States, it presents an entirely different picture. Forty percent of sexually active men are infertile; in its first year on the market, more than one 1 million prescriptions for Viagra were written solely for impotence. Heart disease is the number one killer of men in America, and hypertension is rampant. More than 70 percent of men over age 60 will have prostate problems requiring medication of some kind, and men continue to die on the average eight years before women.

It doesn't present a very healthy picture of the American male, nor does it say much for a health care system that seldom addresses the needs of half of the population. Information is sorely lacking, books are not available, and men seldom, if ever, talk about their needs. Sadly, the holistic healing community has little more to offer men for either their health problems or maintaining well-being (except for anabolic protein powders to build mass) than the conventional medical circles. Something's wrong with this picture.

Helping Men Help Themselves

When I opened my herb store in 1972 in the midst of a lively alternative community in Sonoma County, California, most of my customers were women. They came to buy herbs for themselves, their kids, and sometimes their partners. I can remember the occasional male customer who ventured into the store. He would generally wait until no one else was in the shop, slowly wind his way to the front counter, and begin talking about everything under the sun but the specific problem that had brought him there. I'd find some gentle way to create a space for him to talk about his prostate problems, or herpes, or impotence, or even heartbreak. Sometimes, it was something as simple as a cold or a bad case of poison oak that he was so hesitant to ask help for.

Being young, I figured it had to be that because I was a woman, men weren't as comfortable talking to me. I hadn't yet discovered that men didn't talk about these things to other men either. I also erroneously considered, as many people do, that men don't have the same degree of complexity of physiological function. After all, where were the breasts, the womb, the ability to give birth? I find this rather limited perspective amusing now, and apologize for it, having discovered how complex, marvelous, and cyclic the male system is.

The Complexity of Male Health Care

What is finally being acknowledged is that men's bodies and needs are just as complex as women's, and that they have many concerns surrounding ill health — men just deal differently. Women talk about their problems. They seek help. They turn to other women. Women spend a great deal of time when they are together talking about their feelings, their desires and dreams, their health, and about men. These are not topics that come up much in men's circles. Jobs, sports, politics, and women are often the talk. It's not considered manly to be ill, or worse, to be emotionally or physically in need. It's the "get the job done at all costs" mentality.

One evening my former husband, Karl, was telling me about an exciting football game he played in college. He was the quarterback, had the ball, and was running wildly toward the goal when he was knocked down and severely injured his shoulder. But rather than tell anybody, he played until the end of the game in severe pain with a shoulder practically pulled out of the socket. He was admired by his teammates for his tenacity, and even to this day, many years later, he still tells this story with a mixture of pride and sheepishness, because that shoulder still gives him lots of pain. I find this story interesting because it demonstrates the way men are trained to be, what they pride themselves in and are admired for. Even at their own expense — often at great cost to their bodies, and certainly their feelings — they'll get the job done.

Women foster this attitude in men as much as men do, and may have a greater interest in doing so than we like to admit. It's easy to see the stupidity of sacrificing your body to carry a ball across a mown field. It's easy to get outraged about the ludicrousness of war and the horrors of it. But who benefits when you translate that same attitude to mean "women and children first" at *any* cost?

The Role of Men in Traditional Medicine

It has often been reflected that modern medicine, the Western allopathic model so familiar today, is a perfect heroic system of medicine in which the healer is often the hero. It is typically a male-dominated healing system and is the medical model of choice for emergency situations, for the "cut and stitch" care needed in accidents and life-threatening situations. Author James Green speculates that "today's western, technological, crisis medicine is the male's folkloric tradition in the making."

Designed for war, accidents, acute pain, and critical situations in which heroic measures can be enacted, conventional medicine provides a perfect system of crisis intervention but offers little in the way of preventive health care or medicine that works in accordance with a person's natural process of healing.

Herbalism for Men

At the apprentice programs I offer at my home, Sage Mountain, we always devote a few days to discussing herbal protocols for the reproductive systems of women and men. I will be honest in saying that we generally devote a full two days to women's health, while the topic of men's health is given, at most, a mere half day. Is this discrimination? We could argue that it's because there are more women in the class and a greater percentage of women will seek out herbal health care. Up to this time, that's been true.

Rather than teach the workshop on men's health, I spend some time sharing information on the herbs most often used for men's health problems and highlight some of the major health concerns men have. Then I invite all the men in the class to participate on a panel. The women are invited to ask men questions about health and healing.

In the early years of this course, the women would ask their questions, and before the men had a chance to answer, another woman would answer. There were always lively discussions — usually among the women. The men generally added a comment or two, when it could be squeezed in, but, on the whole, they listened politely. The outcome was that we never did learn much other than what we already knew, and certainly learned nothing from a male perspective.

After a couple of tries with this failed format, we changed the rules. The women were still invited to ask the questions, but they couldn't answer them nor could they offer their perspectives. I learned a lot about men's health listening to the heartfelt responses of these men as they struggled to answer deep and sensitive questions about health, communication, safety, and healing.

Striking the Perfect Balance

Unlike allopathic medicine, herbal medicine offers the supreme preventive and non-crisis-oriented medicine. Herbs build and strengthen the body's natural immunity and defense mechanisms. They nourish the deep inner ecology of our systems on a cellular level. Our bodies know plant medicine simply because we have been evolving with them on this planet for several million years as well as breathing the air they make for us at every moment, eating the food they provide for us, and drinking in the beauty they create around us.

Allopathic and herbal medicine together form a perfect balance for the many health problems facing both men and women today. Men are just discovering the same potential for their own herbal health care that women have been utilizing for years. Herbs like saw palmetto, St.-John's-wort, nettle, and ginseng are finding their way into health care products for men, not as crisis-type medicine, but as preventives. Perhaps as men find ways to explore their own health and healing, they'll have less need for crisis intervention because they will focus on prevention and well-being.

Sharing Different Perspectives

I want to thank you for your patience with my obviously feminine perspective of men's health. I hope it will provide insight and balance, but I must admit I feel a bit like one of the women in my classes on men's health, asking the men their thoughts then proceeding on, without a pause, with my own ideas and opinions.

So, it is my hope as I write this book that it will offer a unique and valuable perspective. I am venturing into a subject that I know well through the men in my life, my male clients, fellow herbal practitioners, and the place of maleness in myself. But I am a guest here, so please excuse me if I'm sometimes clumsy and don't always know the proper protocol. Somewhere, I think, there exists a silent agreement between men and women that we are all venturing into new territory, exploring different ways to be and feel together, and creating a healthier threshold of understanding.

chapter two

Commonsense Guidelines for Good Health

Good health is not a complicated matter. Being in good health doesn't mean you never get sick, or tired, or depressed. But it does mean that you feel hardy most of the time; your body feels fine and your spirits are high. In the words of that wonderful singer, Taj Mahal, "You wake up and morning smiles back at you." Maintaining good health requires excellent daily habits and practices. Preventing, rather than treating, problems is the key to living a long, high-quality life.

Living Healthy

There's no great secret to good health, certainly not the instant pill or cure-all that we're constantly bombarded with by the health and beauty industry. Good health requires simple commonsense practices on a regular basis. Generally, when we become susceptible to illness or are lacking in vitality, it's not due to any great mystery, but to lack of exercise, sleep, good dietary practices, and quality time with friends and family.

Following are the simple guidelines that create radiant vitality. For even more ideas on the practices of healthy living, consult my favorite little book on the topic: *The Art of Good Living*, written by Dr. Svevo Brooks, a naturopathic doctor and athlete.

Exercise is Essential

Men need to exercise. They were not meant to sit at desks all day, not moving their bodies. James Green, author of *The Male Herbal*, feels that lack of exercise is the second most important factor in men's health, or lack of it, in modern society (the first being the lack of bitter herbs — which stimulate and assist digestion — in the diet). Fatigue and ill health are often the result of oxygen-deficient cells. Vigorous physical work is accompanied by an increase in breathing and heartbeat, which causes a rapid exchange of oxygen on a cellular level. The entire body is revitalized and uplifted via the cells.

Mental work, in which so many men are involved today, is far more fatiguing than physical work. The brain requires a greater rejuvenation time than the body, and mental work definitely does not increase the oxygen levels in the body. For good health, exercise daily. Any type of exercise will do, depending on one's individual needs.

Some men respond best to mind-quieting yoga practices, while others are able to "let off steam" in aerobic activities. It's important to realize that the body needs movement every day, and you need to find the kind of activity that works best for you. I might also suggest that you not forgo "life exercise" in lieu of a gym regimen. Be sure to get out and hike, bike, ski, play games, and let your body and spirit interact with the life around you. There's something far more satisfying in stacking a cord of wood than in pedaling a stationary bike.

Maintain a Balanced Diet

Diet is another of those marvelously effective yet simple keys to health and vitality. Eat well-balanced, simple, unadulterated foods. It's not always necessary or even good to follow strict dietary disciplines, but rather follow the laws of healthy eating: Eat food as close to nature as possible, eat what's in season, prepare it simply, chew slowly, and give thanks. For more information on creating health and healing through the foods you eat, see the books listed in Recommended Reading.

Use Herbs Every Day for Health and Vitality

Don't wait until you're sick to use herbs. There is a wonderful variety of herbs that can and should be used daily to enhance wellness. Some of them are listed in chapter 4, but many others, such as horsetail, passionflower, cleavers, chickweed, red clover, and lemon balm, are rich in nutrients that are sustaining to good health and should be used often.

Foods for the Male System

FOOD	BENEFIT
pumpkin seeds	rich in zinc; excellent for the prostate
sesame seeds	calcium-rich; support the nervous system
sesame or tahini butter	calcium-rich
squash seeds	high in zinc; good for the prostate and male glandular system
yogurt	aids digestion; supports the immune system
cultured milks, such as buttermilk	aid digestion; supports the immune system
fresh fruit	excellent source of vitamins, minerals, and fiber
dark green leafy vegetables	excellent sources of minerals, vitamins, and fiber
fish	contain high-quality proteins
chicken	contains high-quality proteins

FOODS TO AVOID

Foods that agitate and exacerbate male health problems when consumed in more than moderate amounts include sugar, alcohol, caffeinated foods (coffee, chocolate, soft drinks), and processed, adulterated foods containing preservatives, food coloring, and artificial flavorings.

I've included several of my favorite male tonic recipes in chapter 5. Make up a pound of the mixture(s) at a time and store in airtight glass jars so they're ready to use. Brew up a quart or two of your favorite herb tea daily. These herb teas not only provide essential nutrients but also help cut back on the consumption of other "less than good for you" drinks. (Need I mention them by name?)

Kegel Exercises

I've yet to meet anyone knowledgeable about reproductive health who doesn't advocate doing kegels on a regular basis for the health of the entire genitourinary system. It's a simple little exercise that was developed in the '40s by Dr. Arnold Kegel, a gynecologist, to help women with urinary problems and bladder control.

Quite by accident, it was discovered that exercising the pubococcygeal muscle on a daily basis not only helped with bladder control, but also enhanced sexual performance, increased circulation to the pelvis, and increased overall health of the reproductive area. Kegels are beneficial for both men and women, and are especially recommended for men with prostate problems, low sexual energy, lack of bladder control, and poor circulation. The wonder of this exercise is that you can do it anywhere, anytime, anyplace: while driving in the car, while sitting reading or watching TV, or while standing in line at the grocery store.

The pubococcygeal muscle is a large, bandlike muscle that runs from the pubic bone to the coccyx. It's the muscle you feel when you squeeze your anus. One way to test its strength is to get up a good flow of urine, then try stopping it midstream. A well-toned pubococcygeal works like a faucet, turning on and off quickly.

To do kegels, first identify the muscles by pulling inward and upward while tightening the anus at the same time. Pull up as hard as you can, hold, relax, and release. It's suggested to start off by doing 10, then 20, 30, and slowly working up to 100 a day. It's guaranteed to make your sex life better (especially if your partner is exercising too).

Yang/Yin: The Theory of Opposites

Throughout this book, I use the terms *yang* and *yin* in reference to certain energetics inherent in all life forms and based on a carefully thought-out Chinese philosophy of opposites.

Yang generally refers to an expansive energy, while yin generally refers to a contractive or inward force. Qualities associated with yang include warm, dry, male, sun, day, fire, light, heaven. The energy moves up and outward, expanding into the world. It is the creative or firm principle.

Qualities associated with yin are cool, moon, night, water, cold, dampness, darkness, female, earth. The energy of what is yin moves downward and inward. It is the receptive or yielding principle.

Men and women, food, movement, art, all of life can be represented in varying degrees by these two principles. A healthy, harmonious life is created by continuously striving for a balance between the opposites of yin and yang, the expansive and the contractive. For a more thorough understanding of these principles and how they apply to diet and health, read Annemarie Colbin's *Food and Healing.*

chapter three

Making and Using Herbal Remedies

Thе single most important factor when purchasing herbs for making remedies is recognizing and obtaining the best quality available. Buy your herbs from reputable companies, companies that have a conscience and that are concerned about both the quality of the products they sell you and the environment. Ask where there herbs come from. Are they organically grown? Are they wildcrafted? If wildcrafted, are they done so ethically, with respect for the environment?

How to Find Good-Quality Herbs

Whenever possible, use your herbs fresh. However, for a variety of reasons, it is not always feasible to get fresh herbs. Dried herbs, if harvested and dried properly, will generally retain all of their medicinal properties. There are few exceptions to this: Chickweed and cleavers really don't dry well and are best fresh, while cascara sagrada and orrisroot must be dried to be used safely.

How do you tell if a dried herb is of good quality? It should look, smell, and taste almost exactly as when it's fresh, and it should be effective. Here are the three guidelines for determining the quality of herbs.

Color

The dried herb should remain almost the same color as when fresh. If you are buying green leaves such as peppermint or spearmint, they should be vivid and bright. If buying blossoms, they should be bright and colorful. For instance, calendula (marigold) should be a bright orange or yellow. Roots, though generally subtle shades to begin with, should remain true to their original color. Goldenseal should be a golden green, echinacea a silvery brown, yellow dock root a yellowish brown. In the beginning, you may not always know what the correct color of a plant should be, but look for liveliness, vibrancy, and deep, strong colors. You will soon develop a knack for knowing.

HOW TO STORE HERBS

Light, heat, air, moisture, and age are the major factors that destroy the essence of herbs. Insects also can be a problem. The ideal storage containers for herbs are glass jars with tight-fitting lids, though other airtight containers work well, too. Store your herbs away from direct light and heat; a cool, dark kitchen closet or pantry is excellent. Herbs stored this way will last for several months or even years.

Smell

Herbs have distinctive odors that serve as effective means of determining quality. They should smell strongly, not necessarily "good." The scent of valerian, for instance, has been compared to dirty socks. Good-quality valerian should smell like *really* dirty socks. Good-quality peppermint will make your nose tingle and your eyes water. Some herbs just smell "green," such as alfalfa. But in that green odor is a freshness and unmistakable vitality. Beautiful, exotic, fragile, sometimes offensive, herbs smell a variety of ways.

Taste

Herbs should have a distinctive fresh flavor. Do not judge them on taste by expecting them to taste good. You will quickly learn that not all medicinal herbs taste good by any stretch of the imagination! So judge taste on potency rather than flavor. Do they taste fresh? Strong? Vital? Distinctive? Do they arouse a distinctive response from your taste buds?

Determining Dosage

Even in conventional (allopathic) medicine, correct dosage is far more arbitrary than we're led to believe. Herbalists are just quicker to admit that determining dosage involves some skill, a healthy touch of "inner knowing," observation, and a bit of guesswork.

In determining proper dosage of an herbal preparation, you must consider the herb itself, what its primary action is, whether it has any toxic side effects, whether it's tonic in its action or a medicine used specifically for a health problem or organ system. Consider the constitution of the person: Is he relatively healthy? Robust or sensitive? Weak or debilitated? And, finally, consider the nature of the imbalance or illness. Is it chronic or acute? Excess or deficient in nature? These factors will help you determine a more accurate dosage, but ultimately, you must trust the wisdom of your own body (or that of the person being treated); listen to what it is telling you. This is often the best advice.

Dosage Chart for Men

Chronic Problems *include long-term imbalances such as hay fever, arthritis, and long-term bronchial problems, which may flare up with acute symptoms periodically. Guidelines for treating chronic problems are as follows:*

TEA	EXTRACTS/ TINCTURES*	CAPSULES/ TABLETS
3–4 cups daily for several weeks	½–1 teaspoon 3 times daily	2 capsules 3 times daily

Acute Problems *are sudden conditions that reach a crisis and need quick attention, such as toothaches, wounds, cuts, and sudden onset of cold or flu. Guidelines for treating acute problems are as follows:*

TEA	EXTRACTS/ TINCTURES*	CAPSULES/ TABLETS
¼–½ cup served throughout the day, up to 3–4 cups	¼–½ teaspoon every 30–60 minutes until symptoms subside	1 capsule every hour until symptoms subside

includes syrups and elixirs

How to Prepare Herbs

The most common methods of preparing herbs for medicinal purposes are tinctures, capsules, and herbal teas. But don't limit yourself. Herbs can be prepared and administered in many creative ways. Syrups and elixirs are a delicious and effective way to down the medicinal properties of herbs. You can also add powdered herbs to food or mix the powders into a paste with honey and spices for a delicious daily tonic.

Some herbs, such as hawthorn and elder, can be prepared as tasty jams and jellies, not a bad way to take medication. And though men are not famous for herbal bathing, it's one of the most relaxing and enjoyable ways to use herbs. When soaking in a warm herbal bath, the pores of the skin, our largest organ of elimination and assimilation, are wide open and receptive. It's like soaking in a giant cup of tea; your entire body reaps the benefits.

Making the Correct Measurements

While many people are converting to the metric system, I've reverted to the Simpler's method of measuring. Many herbalists choose to use this system because it is extremely simple and very versatile. Throughout this book you'll see measurements referred to as "parts": 3 parts sarsaparilla, 1 part Siberian ginseng, 2 parts dandelion root. The use of the word "part" allows the measurement to be determined in relation to the other ingredients. A part is a unit of measurement that can be interpreted to mean cups, ounces, pounds, tablespoons, or teaspoons — as long as you use that unit consistently throughout the recipe. So the formula noted above can be measured as 3 tablespoons sarsaparilla, 3 tablespoons Siberian ginseng, and 2 tablespoons dandelion root. Or, if you want to make medicine in bulk, use cups instead of tablespoons; just keep the relative proportions of each herb consistent.

BUYING VS. MAKING

If making your own herbal products is not your cup of tea, you can go to any natural foods store and purchase ready-made products. Though the choices in ready-made products specifically for men are increasing every day, I would encourage you to at least try your hand at herbal medicine making. Like the great chefs of world-class restaurants, some of the best medicine makers are men. Allow yourself the pleasure of discovering how simple, easy, and effective it is to make herbal medicines.

Making Medicinal Herb Tea

There are whole books on the art of making tea. In fact, I've written many pages myself on this fine subject. But suffice it to say it's probably the easiest preparation you can make in the kitchen. If you've never cooked a thing in your life, trust me, you can make a good cup of medicinal tea. There are two basic methods used for brewing herbs for medicinal purposes, and two auxiliary methods that I'll explain just because they're fun.

Method I: Infusion

Leaves, flowers, and aromatic plants require infusing or steeping as opposed to simmering because they lose their properties more quickly than do roots and barks. Simply boil 1 quart of water per 1 ounce of herb (or 1 cup water to 1 tablespoon of herb). Pour water over the herb(s) and let steep for 30 to 60 minutes. The proportion of water to herb and the required time to infuse varies greatly depending on the herb. Start out with the above proportions and then experiment. The more herb you use and the longer you let it steep, the stronger the brew. Let your taste buds and your senses guide you.

SOME TEA-MAKING TIPS

While every herb is different, here are a couple of tips for making the perfect infusion:

- Let the tea infuse for the length of time necessary to extract the medicinal properties from the herbs. You can tell, because the mixture will taste distinctly herbal.
- Make your tea in quart jars with tight-fitting lids. For a strong tea, let the herbs infuse overnight and strain the next morning. A French coffee press is great for making medicinal teas, but don't use the same one for coffee and herbs; the flavors will mingle. Cover the spout with a towel so as not to let the steam escape; it will carry away many of the vital medicinal properties.

Method II: Decoction

Decoctions are used to make tea from the more tenacious parts of the plant such as roots, barks, and hard seeds or nuts. These plant materials require more direct heat and lower exposure to the heat. Place the herbs in a pot of cold water, cover tightly, bring to a low simmer, and simmer for 30 to 45 minutes. Often, I'll let the herbs sit overnight in the water and strain the next morning.

Solar and Lunar Teas

I often use the energy of the sun and moon when preparing medicinal teas. Never underestimate the powers of these great luminaries. They affect us every day. Why not use that power in your tea? Solar energy is associated with masculine energy. I often make sun teas for men who are seeking to enhance the qualities of the sun in their lives: brightness, sunny disposition, largeness of spirit, warming. The moon is the feminine luminary and is used to enhance dreams, visions, intuition, and the receptive part of oneself.

Solar tea. Place the herbs in a large jar with a tight-fitting lid. Cover with water, then place in direct sunlight and leave exposed to the sun for several hours. If you wish to have a particularly potent tea, prepare first as directed above (see Infusions for leaves and Decoctions for roots) and then allow the sun to work its magic.

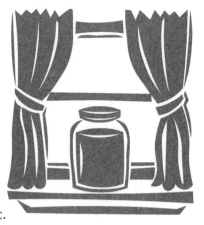

Lunar tea. Place the herbs in a jar or glass bowl, cover with water, and place directly in the path of the moonlight. It's not necessary to place a lid on the container. Leave overnight, then drink the tea first thing in the morning. If you wish a particularly potent tea, prepare first as directed above, depending on whether you're using roots or leaves, then place the tea in the moonlight.

Herbal Capsules

Herbal capsules are many people's favorite way to ingest herbs. They're quick and easy to take as well as being virtually tasteless. But until recently, the herbs contained within capsules were usually very poor quality, with the vital constituents lost through improper heating processes. Most of the capsule containers used were gelatin based, which is difficult to digest and leaves a gummy residue, not to mention that it's a by-product of the slaughter industry.

There has been, however, a transformation in the capsule industry with the recent availability of veggie caps. Plant based, these capsules dissolve quickly and are completely digestible. New cryogenic grinders powder the herbs at sub-zero temperatures, retaining all of the plant constituents. The powdered plants smell and taste fresh and are of far better quality. When buying capsules, buy from those companies that have gone to the extra trouble of ensuring the quality of the product.

USING POWDERED HERBS

Though capsules are quick and easy, powdered herbs can be used in far more creative ways than capsules. Mix them into honey to form a paste, blend them with blender drinks, make candy balls with them. I've included a few of my favorite recipes utilizing powdered herbs in chapter 5.

Making Herbal Capsules

You can easily make your own herbal capsule formulas by placing powered herbs in each side of a size 00 capsule (available at a health foods store) and then joining the two sides. This process is time consuming, although there are inexpensive little capsule machines available that quicken the job. The primary advantages of making your own herbal capsules are that you can customize your herb blend formula and be assured of the quality of the product you're using.

Tinctures

Tinctures are concentrated extracts of herbs. They are taken simply by diluting a few drops of the tincture in warm water or juice. Most tinctures are made with alcohol as the primary solvent or extractant. Though the amount of alcohol is very small, many people choose not to use alcohol-based tinctures for a variety of sound reasons. You can also make effective tinctures using either vegetable glycerin or apple cider vinegar as the solvent, but they are not as strong as alcohol-based tinctures.

Tinctures have a very long shelf life, lasting almost indefinitely, and should be stored in a cool, dark location. Because of their concentration, follow the dosage chart on page 16 carefully.

Instructions for Making Herbal Tinctures

While there are several methods for making tinctures, the traditional or Simpler's method is the one I prefer since it is easy and reliable. All that is required is the herbs, the menstruum (solvent), and a jar with a tight-fitting lid.

Step 1. Chop your herbs finely. I recommend using fresh herbs whenever possible. High-quality dried herbs will work well also, but one of the advantages of tincturing is the ability to preserve the fresh attributes of the plant. Place the chopped herbs in a clean, dry jar.

Step 2. Pour the menstruum over the herbs. *Completely cover* the herbs with the menstruum and then add two to three inches more liquid. If using vegetable glycerin, dilute it first with an equal amount of water. If using vinegar as the menstruum, warm the vinegar before pouring it over the herbs. Warming the vinegar helps facilitate the release of herbal constituents. If choosing alcohol as your solvent, select one that contains 80- to 100-proof alcohol such as vodka, gin, or brandy. Half of the "proof" of the alcohol is the percentage of alcohol in the spirits: 80-proof brandy contains 40 percent alcohol, 100-proof vodka contains 50 percent alcohol. Cover the jar with a tight-fitting lid.

Step 3. Place the jar in a warm place and let the herbs and liquid soak (macerate) for four to six weeks. The longer the time, the better.

Step 4. I encourage the daily shaking of the tinctures during the maceration period. This not only prevents the herbs from packing down on the bottom of the jar, but is also an invitation for some of the old magic to come back into medicine making. Empower your herbal remedies with prayer and song.

Step 5. At the end of the appropriate period of maceration, strain the herbs from the menstruum. Use a large stainless steel strainer lined with cheesecloth or muslin. Reserve the liquid, which is now a potent tincture, and compost the herbs. Rebottle and label.

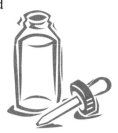

Herbal Syrups

Syrups are among the tastiest of all herbal preparations. They are delicious, concentrated extracts of herbs cooked into a sweet medicine with the addition of honey and/or fruit juice. Maple syrup and vegetable glycerin may be substituted for honey.

Making Herbal Syrups

Although there is more than one method for making an herbal syrup, I have been using this technique for many years. Making the syrup can be a bit time consuming, but this method makes excellent syrups, time after time.

Step 1. Use two ounces of herb mixture to one quart of water. Over low heat, simmer the liquid down to one pint. This will give you a very concentrated, thick tea.

Step 2. Strain the herbs from the liquid. Compost the herbs and pour the liquid back into the pot.

Step 3. To each pint of liquid, add one cup of honey (or other sweetener such as maple syrup, vegetable glycerin, or brown sugar). Most recipes call for two cups of sweetener (a 1:1 ratio of sweetener to liquid). I find it far too sweet for my taste. Aside from flavor, the added sugar helped preserve the syrup when refrigeration wasn't common.

Step 4. Warm the honey and liquid together only enough to mix well. Most recipes instruct cooking the honey and tea together for 20 to 30 minutes longer over high heat to thicken further. It does certainly make a thicker syrup, but I'd rather not cook the living enzymes out of the honey.

Step 5. When finished heating, you may wish to add a fruit concentrate to flavor, or a couple of drops of essential oil such as peppermint or spearmint, or a small amount of brandy to help preserve the syrup and to aid as a relaxant in cough formulas.

Step 6. Remove from the heat and bottle for use. Syrups will last for several weeks, even months, if refrigerated.

Herbal Baths

Most men don't enjoy baths, preferring the quick "in and out" efficiency of the shower. Perhaps this is simply because of the anatomy of modern bathtubs that tend to be small and shallow and don't accommodate the larger male body. While attempting to enjoy the relaxing benefits of an herbal bath, half of the poor fellow is sticking out of the tub freezing! You might consider investing in an old-style clawfoot tub — it's well worth it.

Herbal bathing is worth the effort because it is one of the most relaxing, soothing home treatments for stress, depression, anxiety, and strained, tired muscles. Herbal baths are an excellent way to get the essence of herbs into your body. The warm water opens the pores of the skin, and the herbal nutrients flow in.

The temperature of the water will affect the healing quality of the bath. Cool to tepid water is excellent when trying to lower a fever or normalize the system. A warm bath is relaxing and soothing to the nervous system. Cold water is stimulating and contracting and will firm and strengthen the entire system if you're brave enough to endure.

One last invitation to the bath, for all of you nonbathing males: Aside from your bed, your bathtub may be the most sensuously arousing place in your home, perhaps yet undiscovered. And women usually love to bathe. . . .

How to Make an Herbal Bath

Place a handful of herbs in a cotton bag, nylon sock, or strainer and tie on to the nozzle of the tub. Let the hot water run through it for a few minutes, then release the container into the tub and adjust the temperature of the water. Another method is to prepare a strong herbal tea and add the tea water, after being strained, to the bathwater.

chapter four

The Man's Herbal Medicine Chest

In writing a *materia medica* for men, one is often steered toward those herbs that have a wild reputation for increasing sexual performance, endurance, and stamina. It's interesting, isn't it? Even in herbalism, we create a gender bias. I, too, have included many of the herbs reputed for their "maleness," not as aphrodisiacs per se, but because they are beneficial for their specific toning and revitalizing effects on the male reproductive system. I've also included a number of herbs that strengthen the heart, aid in circulation, and brighten the spirit, and those marvelous tonic herbs that nourish and strengthen the entire system.

Every herb is replete with legends that take us back into ancient times. Though often they seem quaint and antiquated, these stories provide valuable insights into the current uses of the plants. Most of these herbs, being tonic in action, can be used successfully over a long period of time for a variety of purposes. Warnings are given when appropriate.

Listen to Your Body

Reading will fill your head with the wonderful facts and stories about each plant, but herbalism is more than "head" learning. The best possible way to learn about each herb is to experience it. After you've read about it, if it seems like an herb that is appropriate for your situation, try it. The taste, the smell, the effect of the herb on your being is the best

DO YOUR RESEARCH

I've always felt it a requisite when studying herbs to reference *each* herb you're planning to use in at least *three* different herb books. Because herbs are so multifaceted, no one book will give you a complete picture of what it is or what it can do. But reading about the herb in several books will paint a more complete picture for you and give you a broader understanding of its depths and possibilities. For recommended reference books see page 85.

laboratory you have for determining its effectiveness. Women seem to be much more adept at trusting this "knowing." But trust me, the herbs will tell you. They have been communicating with people for thousands of years.

Listen to the wisdom of your body, the feeling of the herbs as you're using them, and the book knowledge you gain as you read and study about them. And don't let your knowing be based on taste alone. Often a very fine herb will have a rather unpleasant flavor. In fact, "rather unpleasant" is a polite understatement of the flavors of some of our best medicinal plants.

Ashwangandha (Withania somnifera)

Parts used: roots

Benefits: An ancient Ayurvedic herb, ashwangandha is referred to in India as the Indian ginseng, and is used very much the way that ginseng is used in Asia. An excellent adaptogenic herb, ashwangandha increases the body's overall ability to adapt to and resist stress. It promotes general well-being and enhances stamina, thus it is popular with athletes. It is both energizing and soothing. It is a classic reproductive tonic and will help restore sexual chi (energy).

Characteristics: Though it's generally grown in India, several friends of mine are successfully growing ashwangandha in the United States. The herb is grown as an annual, and by harvest time, the roots are large and robust.

Suggested uses: Indicated for reduced levels of energy, general debilitation, reduced sexual energy, nervous tension, stress, and anxiety. Ashwangandha is especially useful for sexual problems associated with nervous stress.

Preparation tips: Said to have the smell of a female horse's urine and the stamina of a stallion, ashwangandha isn't your best-tasting herb, though it can be blended with other more flavorful herbs such as ginger, sarsaparilla, and cinnamon to make a suitable tea. In India, the root is powdered and mixed with milk for a classic rejuvenating drink. Try blending it with your favorite chai blend (see recipe on page 57), in a tincture, or in capsule form.

Chaste tree
(Vitex agnus-castus)

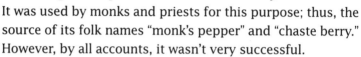

Parts used: berries

History: Named *agnus castus* (chaste) by the Greeks, vitex gained a reputation of calming sexual passions in men. It was used by monks and priests for this purpose; thus, the source of its folk names "monk's pepper" and "chaste berry." However, by all accounts, it wasn't very successful.

Benefits: Vitex is not a true anaphrodisiac. It neither suppresses nor increases libido. Rather, it is a normalizing herb for the reproductive system. Vitex has a stimulating effect on the pituitary gland, which among other functions regulates and normalizes hormone production in both men and women. Because of this, it will either stimulate or suppress sexual expression as necessary.

Suggested uses: Use as a reproductive tonic, for balancing hormones, and for depression and anxiety associated with midlife crisis or middle age.

Preparation tips: Can be prepared in wines, liqueurs, tinctures, and in capsule form. It has a rather hot, spicy flavor not always appropriate for tea. Try it in Chai Hombre, in place of the peppercorns (see page 57).

Damiana *(Turnera aphrodisiaca)*

Parts used: leaves

History: Damiana has a long reputation as an herb of passion and romance. In fact, its botanical name, *aphrodisiaca,* is a sure giveaway. Native to South and Central America, perhaps its Latin origin helps explain its romantic history.

Benefits: Damiana has long been known to strengthen the reproductive systems of both men and women, though it's most often associated with the male reproductive system, and helps replenish diminished sexual vitality. Its nervine and toning properties make it a good general herb for the nervous system as well as a relaxant and antidepressant.

Suggested uses: For diminished sexual vitality, impotence, infertility, nervous exhaustion, anxiety and depression associated with sexual factors, dream therapy, and for muscle and nerve exhaustion.

Preparation tips: Damiana is most often administered in tincture or capsule form. It is also very effective as a tea, but should be blended with other more tasty herbs such as oats and lemon balm because of its unusual flavor. The most delicious way to take it is the famous Damiana Chocolate Love Liqueur (see page 58).

Ginger (Zingiber officinale)

Parts used: root

History: A favorite for its delicious flavor and remarkable qualities, gingerroot has long been honored for its medicinal attributes. One of the most widely used medicinal herbs in modern China, it was first mentioned in the classic *Pen Tsao Ching* (The Classic Book of Herbs) written by emperor Shen Nung around 3000 B.C.

Benefits: Shen Nung valued ginger for much the same reason we do today. An excellent warming herb, ginger promotes circulation and heat to the entire system. I agree wholeheartedly with the ancient Indian proverb, "Every good quality is contained in ginger."

Suggested uses: Ginger is a specific remedy for problems associated with stagnation or congestion in the reproductive system. It is equally valuable for both the male and female systems. It directs blood to the pelvic area and helps relieve pelvic congestion. Ginger is an excellent digestive aid and is as useful as any drug for motion sickness — without the unpleasant side effects.

Preparation tips: Ginger is terrific as a syrup, and good in many dishes. A particularly pleasant way to enjoy your "medicine" is to suck on candied ginger. Another delicious remedy is hot ginger tea served with honey and lemon.

Ginkgo (Ginkgo biloba)

Parts used: leaves, fruits

History: This is certainly one of my favorite herbs, and judging by the number of ginkgo products out there, a number of other people's as well. It is the sole survivor of a large family of plants that dates back over 200 million years.

Benefits: Most of the literature written about ginkgo focuses on is its memory-enhancing qualities and overlooks some of its other outstanding features. One of the best herbs for the circulatory system, it serves as a cardiac tonic by increasing the strength of the arterial walls. It also reduces inflammation in the blood vessels and helps prevent blood clotting that can lead to blocked arteries. Ginkgo promotes blood flow and oxygenation throughout the entire body.

Suggested uses: Ginkgo works to improve mental stability, memory function, and mental vitality by increasing circulation and vasodilation in the cerebral region. It is also an excellent herb for treating vertigo and is an effective remedy for tinnitus, or ringing in the ear. Ginkgo is an antioxidant and is useful against free radicals. It has proven to be an excellent treatment for arterial erectile dysfunction. I have seen ginkgo halt the progression of Alzheimer's disease more effectively than any other substance.

Preparation tips: I recommend the standardized tinctures and capsules that are commercially available, as well as tea and whole-plant tincture. Some studies suggest that ginkgo doesn't break down in water, but I, like the ancients, have found it wonderfully effective as a tea. As a circulatory tea, blend it with hawthorn and lemon balm. As a tea for enhancing memory, it blends well with sage, rosemary, and gota kola. For stress and anxiety, especially when it's mental worry, blend it with oats and nettle.

Ginseng, American
(Panax quinquefolius)

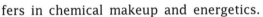

Parts used: roots
Benefits: Connoisseurs of ginseng consider American ginseng the best in the world. Though it has the same tonic, adaptogenic effects as the Asian variety, it differs in chemical makeup and energetics. While Asian ginseng is warming and builds energy and heat in the body, *quinquefolius* is more neutral in its effects and tends to cool and soothe the system, making it a better choice for many American men.
Caution: This is without doubt one of my favorite woodland plants, though it is at risk and difficult to find it in its native habitat these days. Use only organically cultivated or woods-grown ginseng, not wildcrafted varieties.
Suggested uses: For general debilitation, mental clarity, and as a balancing tonic for the entire system. It helps restore energy if used over a period of time, and often is used for anemia and other blood weaknesses. Good for exhaustion and for sexual inadequacy, especially when due to exhaustion or stress.
Preparation tips: Roots should be at least five to six years old (the older the better). Prepare as described below for Asian varieties of ginseng. It has a wonderful bittersweet flavor and can be chewed.

Ginseng, Asian (Panax and related species)

Parts used: roots

History: Considered the "King of All Tonics," ginseng boasts one of the best reputations in the herbal kingdom. Its botanical name, *Panax,* means "cure-all" in Greek, and it has long been considered a male tonic herb. Often the older roots grow in the shape of a man's lower torso.

Benefits: There are many varieties of *Panax* ginseng on the market (American, Asian, Korean, and Chinese). All varieties of ginseng are superior adaptogenic agents that help the body resist a wide spectrum of illness *if* good quality, mature roots are used. When used over a period of time, ginseng restores energy and is especially good for building sexual vitality.

Caution: Though ginseng is an excellent restorative tonic for men, it can sometimes produce too much heat or congestion in the body, especially in those men who tend toward hypertension. I have found ginseng to be counterproductive in "Type A" personalities.

Much of the Asian ginseng imported into or grown in the United States is heavily sprayed with toxic substances. If the roots look large, overly plump, and whitish, be suspicious of the quality. Buy only woods-grown or organically cultivated ginseng, not wildcrafted varieties.

Suggested uses: Rejuvenates the entire nervous system, regenerates frayed or overtaxed nerves, and discourages mood swings and depression. Ginseng restores sexual vitality and rebuilds and restores energy if used over a period of time.

Preparation tips: Roots should be at least five to six years old (the older the better). Ginseng is best used over a period of three to four months. A classic method of preparation is to prepare a strong decoction of a high-quality mature root.

Ginseng blends well with other tonic herbs such as ginger, astragalus, fo-ti, dandelion, burdock, and nettle. I especially enjoy it served with ginger and cinnamon in a chai-type blend (see page 57). Sliced and soaked in honey, the root makes a tasty treat. Because of its good flavor and ease of preparation, I suggest using it in powder form, cooking the roots in soups, and making tea with this granddaddy of all herbs.

THE VERSATILITY OF GINSENG

In Shen Nung's *materia medica* from A.D. 196, ginseng was described as "a tonic to the five viscera: quieting the spirits, establishing the soul, allaying fear, expelling evil effluvia, brightening the eyes, opening the heart, benefiting the understanding, and, if taken for some time, invigorating the body and prolonging life."

However, in the early '80s an American study cited ginseng as the cause of digestive disorders, hypertension, and general malaise. Called GAS (Ginseng Abuse Syndrome), this study baffled longtime users of ginseng. Shortly after the report was released, it was found that the studies had been badly flawed. Much of the herb material being tested was in fact not ginseng at all, but a type of *Rumex* found growing in the prairies of the United States.

Ginseng, Siberian *(Eleutherococcus senticosus)*

Parts used: root, bark

Benefits: Siberian ginseng, often referred to as eleuthero, has almost the same properties as its cousin, *Panax* ginseng. It has a long history of stimulating male virility. It's a superior adaptogenic herb with an impressive range of health benefits. It is commonly used to increase stamina and endurance. Siberian ginseng is also commonly employed as a tonic for the reproductive systems of men.

Characteristics: This variety grows readily and in great abundance. Though not much is cultivated in the United States, this ginseng grows in parks and arboretums in the Northeast.

Suggested uses: Use Siberian ginseng to increase stamina and energy. This herb is also used for suppressed sexual energy due to exhaustion and adrenal depletion. For best results, use over a period of time, several weeks to a few months.

Preparation tips: The flavor of eleuthero is rather inconspicuous and blends well with other tonic and adaptogenic herbs in tea. I also use the powder frequently in foods, candies, and my famous Tonic Male Mash. The roots are an important ingredient in wines and elixirs.

Hawthorn (Crataegus spp.)

Parts used: leaves, flowers, berries, tips of branches

History: Traditionally, the hawthorn tree was planted in or near most herb gardens throughout Europe, and has been revered and surrounded by legend for centuries. Many of the hawthorns my grandmother planted in her yard still bloom.

Benefits: Hawthorn is another of those herbs, along with ginkgo and saw palmetto, that I suggest regularly for men over 45. It is simply the best heart tonic we have, either gently stimulating or depressing the heart's activity as needed. The flowers, berries, tips of branches, and leaves nourish, strengthen, and tone the heart muscle and its blood vessels, and are effective for treating irregular heatbeat and heart palpitations. Hawthorn dilates arteries and veins, allowing blood to flow more freely and releasing cardiovascular constrictions and blockages.

Though not often mentioned in herbal literature, hawthorn is a wonderful remedy for "broken hearts," depression, and anxiety. It is a specific medicine for men who have a difficult time expressing their feelings or who suppress their emotions.

Caution: I have found hawthorn perfectly safe to use when taking heart medication, but if you decide to do so, consult your holistic health care provider or a doctor knowledgeable about the use of herbs.

Suggested uses: This is a tonic herb and should be used over a period of time to be effective. Good for any heart condition, including angina, edema, and heart arrhythmia, and for treating high and low blood pressure and heart palpitations.

Preparation tips: Can be used as a tea, tincture, jam or jelly, and extract. In Europe, where it's a revered and common medicine, it is prepared as jam. Hawthorn berries also make a delicious tea and are often combined with lemon balm and oats for hypertension. The berries, leaves, and flowers are excellent combined with ginkgo leaves as a vascular tonic. For the treatment of high blood pressure, try combining hawthorn leaves, berries, and/or flowers with yarrow and motherwort. Hawthorn is also effective in capsules, though it's so good tasting I would suggest other more tasty herbal preparations. It also makes a good tincture, but again the flavor can be utilized to make elixir and liqueur blends that are exquisite tasting and yet contain all of the nourishing benefits of the plant.

THE STANDARDIZED EXTRACTS DEBATE

There is an argument raging about the advantages and disadvantages of using standardized herbal extracts, which are made through two basic methods. Whole-plant standardization regulates the products made from an herb by determining the amount of its primary active constituent. But no one knows for sure what constituent is the primary active ingredient, and unethical product manufacturers sometimes add synthetic and/or concentrated forms of the chemical in order to match the standardized amount. In the second standardization method, the single active component is removed, giving you one constituent rather than the whole range of plant chemicals.

As we study herbs further, we are reminded that it's the whole plant — the complexity of all the chemicals, the soul, and the spirit of the plant — that makes a medicine active.

Hops *(Humulus lupulus)*

Parts used: strobiles (the leaf bracts surrounding the tiny flowers), pollen

History: Hops is frequently mentioned in literature as a treatment for excessive sexual desire. It was noted that men who worked in the hops fields picking the ripe strobiles reported a significant decrease in sex drive.

Characteristics: The gold-dusted strobiles of hops blossom in the late summer and hang from a golden green vine. These strobiles contain the medicinal parts of the plant.

Benefits: Rich in lupulin, volatile oils, resins, and bitters, hops is a potent medicinal herb highly valued for its relaxing effect on the nervous system. It is especially useful for hypertension and eases tension and anxiety in men, as well as decreasing excessive sexual desire. Hops is one of the most potent bitters, and is excellent as a digestive bitter. It's especially useful for indigestion due to nervous energy and anxiety. Hops is my favorite remedy for insomnia.

Caution: Hops has strong sedative properties; large doses are not recommended for men suffering from depression.

Suggested uses: As a tincture for insomnia, take a couple of hours before bedtime. If you wake up in the middle of the night, take several more large dropperfuls diluted in a bit of warm water. To aid in balancing excessive sexual drive, use ½ teaspoon of the tincture diluted in warm water three to four times a day. As a digestive aid, make your own digestive bitters by combining hops with other bitter herbs such as gentian, dandelion root, and yellow dock, and make a tincture. Take ½ teaspoon of the tincture before meals.

Preparation tips: Hops is extremely bitter. Nothing really disguises the taste well, so hops is generally tinctured or encapsulated. It is also a fine medicine when made into beer, serving as both a sedative and digestive bitter. Be sure the beer is of high quality, or grow the hops and make your own brew.

For insomnia, I prefer mixing hops and valerian tinctures. As a digestive aid you can mix hops with mugwort, motherwort, artichoke leaf, or any of the other digestive bitters.

Kava-kava *(Piper methysticum)*

Parts used: root

History: Native to Polynesia, Melanesia, and Micronesia, kava has been highly revered for hundreds of years in its native cultures. It played an important part in every cere- mony, and was served at most social functions, celebrations, inaugurations, and meetings. The old saying is, "There can be no hate in the heart when one has kava."

Benefits: Has the unique ability to relax the body while awak- ening the mind. It produces a sense of relaxation and at the same time heightens awareness and makes you feel brighter.

Suggested uses: Primarily known for its relaxant properties, kava helps reduce tension, anxiety, and stress. Its analgesic properties help alleviate pain.

Caution: Kava can be overused and abused. Too much kava can make you nauseated, induce unconsciousness, and affect your driving ability. There have already been several cases of people arrested for driving "under the influence" who were actually not drunk, but had overindulged on kava.

Preparation tips: The unique flavor may take some getting used to. Don't be alarmed the first time you try it; it will numb the tongue and create tingling sensations throughout the mouth. These sensations are temporary and are caused by a particular chemical substance in kava called kavalactones.

I generally prefer kava as a tea or punch. Prepare a strong tea; add cinnamon, ginger, and cardamom for flavor. Let the tea sit several hours or overnight, then strain. Add pineapple juice and coconut milk for flavor and serve chilled.

Kava is available as tincture, extract, and capsules. The tincture is a quick, effective, and handy form to use. It is helpful in those times of stress when you need a quick relax- ant, something that helps put the world in perspective. Cap- sules are effective for long-term stress and anxiety.

Licorice (Glycyrrhiza glabra)

Parts used: roots

Benefits: This sweet root is an outstanding tonic herb for the endocrine system and is specific for the reproductive systems of both men and women. The constituents in licorice are similar to the natural steroids in the human body. This herb has a marked positive effect on the adrenal glands and is one of the best herbs we have for adrenal exhaustion, a possible cause of midlife crisis in men.

Licorice is also highly regarded as a remedy for the respiratory system and is used as a soothing demulcent and anti-inflammatory. It's a longtime favorite for coughs, sore throats, and bronchial inflammation, and is particularly beneficial for those who suffer from debilitating and wasting diseases.

Caution: Though there are many warnings against using licorice, it must be remembered that licorice is one of the most widely prescribed herbs in the world and there are very few cases of toxicity reported due to its use. However, licorice is not recommended for individuals who have high blood pressure or edema. People who are on heart medication also should use licorice in only moderate amounts; check with your holistic health care provider before using licorice in combination with heart medication.

Suggested uses: For adrenal exhaustion, tiredness, and fatigue, drink two to three cups of licorice tea a day blended with wild yam, sarsaparilla, burdock root, and sassafras. Licorice is often made into cough syrups for sore throats, mixed with pleurisy root and elecampane for deep-seated bronchial inflammation, and combined with marsh mallow root for digestive inflammation and ulcers. It can be used in tincture and capsules, as well.

Preparation tips: Due to its sweetness, licorice is often used in a blend to flavor other herbs and to alleviate unpleasant symptoms caused by the action of harsher herbs. It has a rich mucilaginous consistency and adds a soothing quality to any syrup or tea it's mixed with. I use licorice powder to flavor other herbal powders and then roll them into tasty little pills and balls.

Muira puama (Ptychopetalum olacoides, Liriosma ovata)

Parts used: bark

History: Native to Brazil, muira puama's use as an aphrodisiac has spread throughout South America, into Europe, and is slowly being "discovered" in the United States. It is a favorite remedy of men who are unable to attain or maintain an erection.

Benefits: This may well be one of the best-kept herbal secrets for impotence and depressed sexual activity. The herb is often referred to as "potency wood" and has a long-standing reputation as a powerful aphrodisiac and nervine. Its mode of action is unknown at this time, but it seems to have no side effects. It is used to treat dysentery, diarrhea, and other diseases for which a strong astringent is indicated.

Caution: Muira puama is considered a tonic herb without any harmful side effects when used in therapeutic dosage. However, there is very little known about this herb, so be mindful as you use it. If you note any undesirable side effects, discontinue immediately.

Suggested uses: Works as a tea, tincture, or in capsule form. Take ½ to 1 teaspoon of the tincture twice daily as a reproductive tonic for several weeks. It can be used in more frequent doses before lovemaking. If in capsule form, the general dosage would be two capsules three times daily. For tea, muira puama is most often combined with other herbs and drunk one cup at a time, three to four times daily.

Preparation tips: Muira puama is often combined with Siberian ginseng, ashwangandha, and circulatory herbs such as ginkgo and hawthorn to help build reproductive health and vitality.

Nettle *(Urtica dioica)*

Parts used: leaves, seeds, roots

Characteristics: The tips of the nettle plant in early spring and summer are superior, though I've eaten them throughout the season. If you have a stand of nettles nearby, it is good practice to trim them constantly throughout the season so they will keep producing those tasty tops until fall.

Benefits: This is the stinging nettle that farmers despise, hikers hate, and children learn to deplore. But herbalists around the world fall at the feet of this green goddess/green man herb. It is a vitamin and mineral factory, rich in iron, calcium, potassium, silicon, magnesium, manganese, zinc, and chromium, as well as a host of others. It activates metabolism by strengthening and toning the entire system. Nettle is a wonderful endocrine system tonic and is used to strengthen both the reproductive system and weak kidneys. It is indicated for liver problems and is also excellent for treating allergies and hay fever. All this and it tastes good too.

Suggested uses: Use in tea form as a tonic for reproductive vitality. Nettle is superior for any liver disorder when used in tea, tincture, or capsule form. Freeze-dried capsules are one of the best ways to use nettle for allergies and hay fever. For urinary health, drink several cups of nettle tea combined with dandelion greens, a combination especially useful for edema.

Preparation tips: Nettle has a rich green flavor and lends itself well to tea blends. Combine it with green milky oat tops and raspberry leaf to combat reduced energy and sexual dysfunction. For liver disorders and congestion, mix with burdock root. For urinary disorders or water retention, combine with dandelion greens. When combined with saw palmetto and made into a tincture, it is excellent for decreasing prostate enlargement.

Ryan Drum, herbalist and wildcrafter extraordinaire, suggests the seeds are among the best and most nourishing of herbal stimulants. In addition, the roots traditionally have been steamed and eaten, though most people ignore them in favor of the tender tops. Try the tops in place of spinach in spanikopita (Greek spinach pie) or with feta cheese and olive oil. You must make sure, however, that the nettle has been properly cooked or you're likely to get pricked while eating it. Nettle can be steamed and served as a green.

Oats *(Avena sativa, A. fatua)*

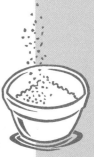

Parts used: green milky tops, seeds, stalks. *Avena sativa* is the cultivated variety; *A. fatua* is the wild version.

Benefits: Oats are among the best tonic herbs for the nervous system and are a superior cardiac tonic. Every man who finds himself overworked, stressed, and anxious, or who has irritated and inflamed nerve endings due to burns or hemorrhoids should include oats in his daily health program. Oats are one of the principal herbal aids used for convalescing after a long illness. They help to soothe irritation from nicotine and other chemical withdrawals. Oats provide energy by increasing overall health, vitality, and stamina. Oat tops are exceptionally rich in silica, calcium, and chromium and are one of the highest terrestrial sources of magnesium. The stalks of oats, though not as rich in minerals as the milky green tops, are also medicinal.

Suggested uses: To treat nervous system disorders, depression and anxiety, low sexual vitality, irritability, and urinary incontinence. Oatmeal is often included as a healing agent in diets for people with poor digestion or inflammation of the digestive tract, or who are weak and debilitated and can't hold food in.

Preparation tips: We're used to thinking of oats in the classic form of oatmeal. But to herbalists, oatmeal is for breakfast, while the delicious oat tops are for tea. They can be combined with lemon balm and passionflower for a good nervine, with valerian for a good sleep aid, or with digestive bitters for any liver or digestive upset. Oats (both the meal and the non-ripened milky tops) make one of the most soothing herbal baths for nervous stress and irritated, itchy skin. (Add several drops of lavender oil for an especially relaxing experience.)

Pumpkin (Cucurbita pepo and related species)

Parts used: seeds

Benefits: Because of their high zinc content, pumpkin seeds have a reputation for being a nonirritating and valued treatment for benign enlargement of the prostate gland. A cytotoxic compound also makes them valuable in the treatment of cancer-induced prostate enlargement. Men who have cuts and wounds that don't heal readily should use pumpkin seeds; they can help those little nicks and scratches heal much more quickly.

Suggested uses: Pumpkin seeds contain bitter compounds that make them one of the most well-known anthelmintics (antiparasitic). Use to improve prostate health. The seeds are also rich in phytosterols, anti-inflammatory agents that make them particularly beneficial in conjunction with pygeum and saw palmetto for the prostate.

Preparation tips: Keep a bowl handy and munch on pumpkin seeds throughout the day. They are excellent added to trail mix and can be sprinkled on salads or in soups and casseroles. Eat up to ¼ cup daily for prostate health and zinc deficiency. Any pumpkin seeds will do, but those of *Cucurbita pepo* are most commonly sold commercially.

Pygeum (Pygeum africanum)

Parts used: bark

History: Used in Africa for centuries for male health, prostate enlargement, and impotence and infertility, pygeum was only introduced into the European and Western herbal medical field in the late 1800s. Little information on this amazing herb is found in early literature.

Characteristics: A folk medicine from Africa, pygeum is a beautiful, large evergreen tree that can reach a height of more than 100 feet. It has startling white flowers and red berries. The medicine comes from the dark, fissured bark.

Benefits: Pygeum is one of the most popular herbs in Europe for the treatment of benign prostatic hyperplasia (BPH), because it promises to reverse the condition, not just control the symptoms. Pygeum also reduces cholesterol levels that have been found to contribute to BPH. It is used to treat enlarged prostate, inflammation, edema, infertility and impotence, and sterility when due to insufficient prostate secretions.

Suggested uses: Combine with saw palmetto or pumpkin seeds to treat prostate enlargement, inflammation, and edema. Pygeum has a different, though complementary mode of action from saw palmetto; so this combination is helpful for many men with congested prostate glands or BPH.

Caution: Pygeum is threatened in its native range due to habitat destruction and overharvesting by lumber, pharmaceutical, and herbal companies; only commercially farmed pygeum should be bought.

Preparation tips: Traditionally, pygeum bark was powdered and mixed with warm milk. Sometimes other spices were used to flavor this drink. It is primarily available in capsules and extracts in the United States, seldom in raw bulk form.

THE MAN AS HERBALIST

More women have been attracted to the study of herbs than men, though I suspect this has to do with the fact that herbalism has not been considered a means toward a viable income, rather than a lack of interest from men. Men more often make decisions on what they will do in life based on income potential and their ability to support a family, rather than their dreams of what they'd like to do. As herbs gain in popularity in this country and job opportunities open, we're seeing a corresponding interest from the male population.

Red Raspberry *(Rubus idaeus)*

Parts used: leaves, roots, berries

Benefits: One of raspberry's best-kept secrets is that it has the same tonic effects on men as it does on women. It is a highly nourishing reproductive tonic, providing nutrients that tone and strengthen the genitourinary system. One of the richest sources of iron, raspberry is used to replenish iron-poor blood and is often combined with nettle for anemia and related low energy levels. Raspberry is also a rich source of niacin and among the richest sources of manganese, a trace mineral that is used by the body to produce healthy connective tissue such as bone matrix and cartilage. Manganese is also an important factor in energy metabolism.

Suggested uses: Use as a nutritive tonic when energy is low, when recovering from illness, and at times when an endocrine tonic is needed. Blended with nettle, it is one of the best herbal combinations for anemia. Due to its organic acid content (i.e., malic and citrus), raspberry has astringent actions and is useful for diarrhea, dysentery, and bleeding.

Preparation tips: The leaf is quite tasty and is generally served as a tea. Drink several cups a day of the infusion to experience its toning effects. It can also be blended with other reproductive tonic herbs and made into a tincture to be used daily. The berries are also medicinal and delicious. Use them to make cordials to toast the gods.

Sarsaparilla *(Smilax officinalis* and related species)

Parts used: roots, rhizomes

History: A native of Central and South America, sarsaparilla was brought to Europe in the fifteenth century as a cure for syphilis.

Benefits: A wonderful aromatic root tonic that is effective as a cleanser or "blood purifier" for the genitourinary system, liver, and gallbladder. Because of its cleansing action, it is often used in formulas to treat skin conditions. The roots are rich in steroidal saponins that provide the building blocks necessary for the body to produce steroidal hormones. It is very rich in trace minerals, primarily selenium and zinc.

Suggested uses: Skin conditions such as psoriasis, arthritis and rheumatism, hormonal imbalances, low energy, poor elimination, and sluggish liver can all be treated with this versatile herb.

Preparation tips: I usually prepare sarsaparilla as a tea because of its rich, wonderful vanilla-like flavor. It adds that classic root beer taste to teas and is wonderful to blend with sassafras, birch bark, dandelion root, and echinacea for a super immune formula that's delicious. Add a pinch of stevia for sweetness.

Sassafras (Sassafras albidum)

Parts used: bark, root bark (the best part of the plant, but one has to dig up the sassafras to get the root bark)

History: This has long been one of my favorite herbs for flavoring teas, especially teas made from roots and barks. It was traditionally the main ingredient in old-fashioned "root beers," tonic drinks that were made from roots and barks for seasonal cleansing.

Benefits: Sassafras is cleansing to the entire system and stimulating for congestion in the liver and gallbladder. It has a grounding (yang) action and is often associated with the male system. A powerful astringent, it can be used externally for insect bites and internally for diarrhea and dysentery. I find it to be one of the best herbs for enhancing the flavor and healing properties of male tonic drinks.

Suggested uses: Male hormonal imbalances, liver congestion, diarrhea, skin disorders, and disruptions in the genitourinary system can be treated with sassafras.

Caution: Sassafras is not mentioned often or used in teas anymore, not because it isn't effective or safe, but because it's currently illegal to use for internal purposes. In the 1970s safrole, a highly toxic chemical constituent, was isolated, extracted with chemical solvents (it's not water soluble) and tested on laboratory rats. It was found, not surprisingly, that in large amounts it produced carcinogenic cells in the rats. No human case of cancer from sassafras has ever been reported. The soft drink industry, which up to that time had been using pure sassafras extracts for flavoring root beer, was forced to substitute synthetic chemicals. (Is that better for us?) Interestingly, the southeastern United States, where sassafras has been drunk as a traditional folk remedy, has the lowest rate of throat cancer in the country. I continue to use it because I know it's a valuable, safe, and effective herb, although regulations prevent me from using it in my commercial formulas, and I don't recommend it to my clients (for ethical reasons) unless they request it.

Preparation tips: Sassafras is water soluble and is quite delicious as tea. It can also be made into tasty elixir and tonic brews.

Saw Palmetto (Serenoa serrulata and S. repens)

Parts used: berries

History: Though long used by the native people of the subtropical coast of North America, saw palmetto's popularity has risen rapidly in recent years.

Benefits: Simply the best remedy for inflammation of the prostate gland. It is tonic in action and serves as an effective diuretic and relaxant. Its fatty fruit is one of the few Western herbs that is anabolic; it encourages weight gain and bulk by strengthening and building body tissue. As a tonic herb, it can be taken on a regular basis to strengthen the urinary and endocrine systems and to prevent future problems with the prostate gland. Why wait?

Nicknamed the "plant catheter," saw palmetto has the ability to strengthen the neck of the bladder and to reduce enlarged prostate glands. It reduces many of the problems associated with an enlarged prostate gland: dribbling urine;

Though saw palmetto isn't a cure for prostate cancer, it may be a preventive. And it's certainly wise to use it as part of a holistic treatment program for prostate cancer. Many allopathic doctors now recommend it as part of their treatment protocol. Prostate cancer is generally very slow growing, easily monitored, and the latest findings suggest that men live the same amount of time with or without the surgery, but have much greater discomfort with the surgery. Often the recommendation is managing the cancer through the use of herbs and diet, rather than surgery.

slow, painful urination; the need to urinate several times during the night; and incomplete urination, which can lead to low-grade cystitis.

Suggested uses: Use to treat prostatitis, low energy due to anabolic stress, cystitis, bladder malfunctions, prostate cancer, and to build weight and bulk.

Preparation tips: Saw palmetto has a fatty, pungent flavor that is hard to get down and hard to disguise. I don't know of many men who enjoy the flavor of this herb in tea. It's usually available in tincture form where the fatty acids are well suspended. It can be used in capsules as well, but they should be fresh and of good quality because the fats in saw palmetto turn rancid quickly.

Valerian (*Valeriana officinalis* and related species)

Parts used: roots

History: Valerian has been highly regarded as an herbal medicine for centuries. Hildegard von Bingen, a famous German abbess/herbalist, used it as a sedative in the twelfth century. In the 1500s the great herbalist Gerard claimed it to be one of the most popular remedies of his time. Today, in spite of its distinct and somewhat offensive odor, valerian continues to be one of the most popular medicinal herbs used in the world.

Benefits: One of the most potent herbs known for the nervous system, valerian is powerful, safe, and very effective. Its name is derived from the Latin word *valere,* "to be well," "be strong." In Europe, where it has been used for centuries, it is used in hundreds of over-the-counter drugs and is relied on primarily as a medicine for stress and tension.

Suggested uses: There is no finer herb than valerian for men who suffer from stress, insomnia, and nervous system disorders. Though potent, it is perfectly safe to use and is not addictive. Valerian is effective both as a long-term nerve tonic and as a remedy for acute problems such as headaches and pain. Valerian has powerful tonic effects on the heart and is often recommended in combination with hawthorn berries for high blood pressure and irregular heartbeat.

Caution: Though generally considered a safe, nontoxic herb, valerian will act as an irritant in some of the people who use it. If you become further agitated and restless after using valerian, discontinue use and consider yourself in that rare 5 percent of the population that can't tolerate this herb.

Preparation tips: Some herbalists prefer the fresh violet-scented roots; others claim the medicinal properties are stronger in the dried roots that smell like dirty socks. It's a personal preference. Don't decoct these roots, as they are rich in aromatic oils (thus the odor). They should be infused only. Though water soluble, most people don't prefer to take their valerian in tea form. It's usually consumed either in tincture or in capsules.

DOSING VALERIAN PROPERLY

Don't be afraid to take adequate amounts of this herb. Begin with low dosages and increase until you feel its relaxing effects. Valerian is nonaddictive, non-habit-forming, and will not make the user sleepy or groggy unless large amounts are consumed. Too much valerian in the system is noted by either a "rubberlike" feeling in the muscles — as if they are *too* relaxed — or a feeling of heaviness. Cut back the dosage so that you feel relaxed, but alert.

Wild Yam *(Dioscorea villosa)*

Parts used: rhizomes, roots

Benefits: A primary source of material for steroid production and also serves as a hormone precursor, thereby aiding the proper function of the reproductive system. Wild yam contains bitter compounds that help tone the liver and increase bile flow. It is one of my favorite herbs for liver congestion and inflammation. It's especially indicated for men who store excess heat (yang) in their bodies or have high blood pressure and is also useful for frayed nerves, musculoskeletal inflammation, and smooth-muscle cramps.

Suggested uses: Treat liver congestion, high blood pressure, hormonal imbalances, muscle cramps and spasms, arthritis, and other injuries to the joints with wild yam.

Caution: Oddly, one sometimes finds wild yam listed as a natural birth-control agent, though it is more often used to promote fertility. Wild sources of this plant are under siege, and some varieties of wild yam are highlighted on the United Plant Savers At-Risk list (see page 89 for more information). Use only cultivated varieties.

Preparation tips: Wild yam is bitter and not often prepared in tea, but is tolerable when blended with other herbs. Often used as a tincture or in capsules, I like to mix the powdered wild yam with other tonic herbs, add cardamom and cinnamon powder to taste, and mix into a paste with honey and rose water.

Yohimbe *(Pausinystalia yohimbe* and *Corynanthe yohimbe)*

Parts used: inner shavings of the bark

History: Yohimbe has a long history of use in its native Africa, where it is primarily used as a potent aphrodisiac and stimulant.

Benefits: I include this herb with some trepidation. Yohimbe is an exciting herb, but it's very potent, potentially harmful, and has a long list of side effects if used improperly. Even in moderate doses it can be overstimulating. It acts both as a central nervous system stimulant and as a mild hallucinogen. Yohimbe stimulates blood flow to the erectile tissue. Yohimbine hydrochloride, a product sold by pharmaceutical companies, is a prescription drug used for treating erectile dysfunction.

Suggested uses: Use cautiously to increase libido, for sexual stimulation, and to treat erectile dysfunction.

Caution: Yohimbe is a monamine oxidase inhibitor (MAOI) and should be used with caution. Do not use yohimbe in combination with sedatives, tranquilizers, antihistamines, narcotics, or large quantities of alcohol. People with kidney disorders, cardiovascular disorders, diabetes, or abnormal blood pressure or blood sugar should not use yohimbe.

Preparation tips: The traditional way to prepare yohimbe is to bring two cups of water to a boil. Add one ounce of yohimbe bark to the boiling water and allow to boil for no more than four minutes. Turn the heat on low and simmer slowly for an additional 20 minutes. Strain, and sip slowly about one hour before desired effect. For a stronger, more effective drink, add 1,000 mg of ascorbic acid (vitamin C) to the brew. The vitamin C reacts with the alkaloids to form yohimbine and yohimbiline ascorbates, more soluble and more active forms of yohimbe. Do not use over a long period of time.

chapter five

Formulas
Especially for Men

T hese are some of my favorite formulas. They are strong, invigorating, and flavorful. Most are tonics and are best used on a daily basis, but each of them can be used as a medicinal and incorporated into health programs. I've provided recipes here for you to try, but you need not follow them to the T. Be creative and have fun with the recipes; you can alter the formulas and flavors to suit yourself. Experimentation might lead to an even better formula!

Fertility & Potency Syrup

This formula has a reputation for increasing virility in men and helping with fertility (if not due to structural causes). It is a tonic formula and needs to be used over a period of three to six months.

1 ginseng root	½ ounce raspberry leaf
½ ounce saw palmetto berries	1 ounce damiana
	1 ounce nettles
1 ounce ashwangandha	1–2 cups honey (to taste)
½ ounce wild yam root	1 cup fruit concentrate
2 ounces muira puama	(available in natural
2 quarts water	foods stores)
2 ounces oats (milky green tops)	½ cup brandy (optional, but will help preserve syrup)

1. Combine ginseng, saw palmetto berries, ashwangandha, wild yam, and muira puama with water. Decoct slowly as instructed on page 19 over low heat until liquid has been reduced to 1 quart. Keep the lid slightly ajar so that some of the steam can evaporate.

2. Turn the heat off, but don't strain. While water is still at its hottest, add oats, raspberry leaf, damiana, and nettles. Let the herbs sit overnight with the lid tightly on.

3. The next day, strain the herbs through a fine-mesh strainer lined with muslin or cheesecloth. Add honey to taste, fruit concentrate, and brandy. Store in refrigerator. Take 2–4 tablespoons daily for 3–6 months. 🌿

Long Life Elixir (For the Sage in Your Life)

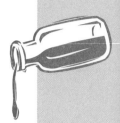

This is by far one of my all-time favorite recipes. It's an herbal tonic that builds strength and vitality, and though it can be used by both sexes, it is predominantly a masculine yang-type tonic and was formulated especially for men.

This recipe invites your creativity; in fact, it yearns for it. Truthfully, I've never followed the exact recipe twice myself.

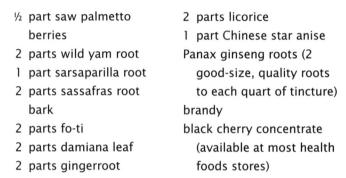

½ part saw palmetto berries
2 parts wild yam root
1 part sarsaparilla root
2 parts sassafras root bark
2 parts fo-ti
2 parts damiana leaf
2 parts gingerroot
2 parts licorice
1 part Chinese star anise
Panax ginseng roots (2 good-size, quality roots to each quart of tincture)
brandy
black cherry concentrate (available at most health foods stores)

1. Make an herbal tincture with the herbs and brandy, as instructed on page 22. Let the mixture sit for 6–8 weeks; the longer the better.

2. Strain. To each cup of liquid add ½ cup black cherry concentrate. Be sure this is a fruit concentrate, not a fruit juice. Shake well, and rebottle. Your elixir is ready for use, although I often put the ginseng roots back in the rebottled tincture. A standard daily dose is about ⅛ cup per day. Serve in a fine little goblet and sip as an aperitif. Try sipping it with your sweetie before a sensuous night.

"ELIXIR FOR THE GODS"

The name Long Life Elixir came about because the first time I made it I stored it in an antique glass bottle that had engraved upon it the Tree of Life and the words LONG LIFE. The name seemed fitting and has stuck. That first jar, brewed so many years ago, went to James Green, author of *The Male Herbal,* who said upon first tasting it, "Its flavor and culinary presence brings to mind words such as 'exquisite' and 'elixir for the gods.'"

Energy Balls

This special, high-powered food supplement is delicious and easy to make. Though there are many "super food bars" on the market, they are expensive and generally not as good as what you can make at home. Try these; they contain nutrients essential to the yang male energy system. They are energizing, restorative, and formulated to build and renew the male reproductive system when used over time. Be sure the herbs are finely powdered or else you'll be picking out little chunks of nonchewable roots.

1 part ginseng powder
2 parts eleuthero (Siberian ginseng) powder
3 parts pumpkin seeds, powdered
½ part spirulina or Super Blue Green Algae®
1 part ginkgo or gotu kola powder
1 cup sesame butter (tahini)
½ cup honey
½ cup crushed almonds
Coconut, cocoa powder, raisins, chocolate or carob chips, and granola for flavor
Carob powder or powdered milk

1. Combine powdered herbs and mix well.

2. Combine the sesame butter and honey, mixing to form a paste. If you want your Energy Balls to be sweeter, add more honey.

3. Add enough of the powdered herbs to thicken, then add the almonds and the flavoring additions. Thicken to desired consistency with carob powder or powdered milk. Roll into walnut-size balls. Eat two Energy Balls daily.

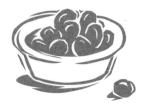

Good Life Wine

This aromatic herbal wine should be served as a tonic. It can be taken in small dosages of ¼ cup daily to promote health and well-being.

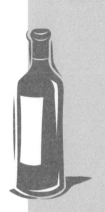

- 1 good-quality medium-size ginseng root
- 4 astragalus roots
- 1 ounce fo-ti
- 1 ounce ashwangandha root
- 2 tablespoons cardamom seeds (crushed)
- 1 ounce damiana leaf
- 2 tablespoons Chinese star anise
- a couple of cloves for flavor
- a pinch of gingerroot for flavor
- 1 quart good-quality wine

1. Place herbs in a largemouthed canning jar and pour wine over the mixture. Cover and let it sit for 3–4 weeks in a warm place in the kitchen.

2. Strain and rebottle into the original wine bottle. The ginseng root can be sliced and added back to the wine. ✱

Male Toner Tea

A flavorful, well-balanced tea especially formulated for the male system, this used to be my personal favorite and was one of the best-selling blends of the early Traditional Medicinal line. However, the FDA ordered us to remove the sassafras due to questions about its safety (see page 45). I never felt it was as good after. You get to choose: sassafras or no? Adjust the flavors as you please.

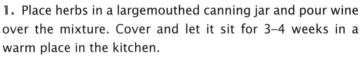

- 1 part ginseng (you can use prince ginseng, Asian, or American varieties)
- 1 part eleuthero (Siberian ginseng)
- 1 part licorice
- 1 part muira puama
- 1 part cinnamon
- ¼ part ginger
- 3 parts sarsaparilla
- 3 parts sassafras
- 1 part wild yam
- ⅛ part orange peel
- 1 part burdock root

Prepare a decoction as directed on page 19. Drink 3–4 cups daily. ✱

Male Vital-a-Tea

A nourishing and delicious formula, Vital-a-Tea is formulated for its high vitamin and mineral content. Drink several cups a day if feeling exhausted and depleted. You'll experience its restorative properties within a few days.

1 part damiana	3 parts ginkgo
2 parts nettle	4 parts hawthorn berries
4 parts oats (milky tops and stalks)	2 parts raspberry leaf
	a pinch of stevia
3 parts lemon balm	a handful of hibiscus

Prepare an infusion as instructed on page 18. Drink 3–4 cups daily. 🐾

Ginseng Tonic Tea

I met Nam Singh many years ago when he was still quite a young man. I knew the minute I met him that I was in the presence of a "master." Of African-American descent, Nam was raised in a Taiwan monastery by his elderly grandfather. Nam was instructed early in the arts of tai chi, Chinese herbal medicine, and acupuncture, and is an amazing practitioner today. Now, in his late 40s, Nam still looks 25. I think he's on his way to becoming one of those ageless sages.

Nam taught me most of what I know about Asian ginseng, and also instructed me how to prepare it using a ceramic ginseng cooker. These double boilers, specially made for preparing ginseng, can be quite ornate and beautiful works of art. It's also possible to pick up inexpensive ones in most Chinese herb stores, but if you can't find one, a regular double boiler will do.

> 1 large, well-aged ginseng root
> water

Place the root in the cooker and cover with water. Tie the cooker shut, then place it in another pan filled with water. Cook over low heat for 6–8 hours. Strain, and drink all of the resulting liquid. It is very potent, to say the least. 🐾

USING GINSENG FOR GOOD HEALTH

Nam Singh recommends fasting for three days prior to drinking the ginseng tea and for three days after. In China the people prefer to use ginseng in this fashion, taking it once or twice a year rather than consuming it daily, as is often done in this country. He also uses it in soups and broths, thus employing it as both a medicine and a food. Prince ginseng, small rootlets that are a distant relative of the ginseng family, is also used in cooking and as an addition to daily tonic teas.

Chai Hombre

A robust, spicy herbal blend originating in India, Nepal, and Tibet, there are literally thousands of different recipes for chai. Following is a chai blend especially formulated for men. It has some of the traditional chai herbs, but added are a number of herbs for male health. Serve it hot or chilled with frothy steamed milk. You can easily make steamed milk at home with an inexpensive device that is available in most kitchen shops.

6 slices fresh gingerroot, grated
4 whole cloves
2 teaspoons cardamom, crushed
3 tablespoons cinnamon chips (or 1 stick broken into small pieces)
6–8 black peppercorns
1 tablespoon sliced ginseng root
1 tablespoon sliced licorice root
1 tablespoon sliced fo-ti
5 tablespoons black tea leaves
6 cups water
honey
steamed milk (can be soy or rice milk)
nutmeg or cinnamon

1. Gently warm herbs and water in a covered saucepan for 10–15 minutes. Do not boil.

2. Strain the mixture into a warmed teapot and add honey to taste. Pour into a large cup, add a generous heap of steamed milk, and sprinkle with nutmeg or cinnamon.

Damiana Chocolate Love Liqueur

When you need that something extra on that oh-so-special night, try this blend from the love goddess herself, Diana DeLuca. This stuff is dangerously lip-smacking good — and daringly easy to prepare. Prepare it ahead of time and serve it at the beginning of a hot date. A variety of other herbs can be added to the basic Damiana Liqueur recipe.

> 1 ounce damiana leaves (dried)
> 2 cups vodka or brandy
> 1½ cups spring water
> 1 cup honey
> vanilla extract
> rose water
> chocolate syrup
> almond extract

1. Soak damiana leaves in vodka or brandy for 5 days. Strain; reserve the liquid in a bottle.

2. Soak the alcohol-drenched leaves in the spring water for 3 days. Strain and reserve the liquid.

3. Over low heat, gently warm the water extract and dissolve the honey in it. Remove the pan from heat, then add the alcohol extract and stir well. Pour into a clean bottle and add a dash of vanilla and a touch of rose water for flavor. Let it mellow for one month or longer; it gets smoother with age.

4. To each cup of damiana liqueur, add ½ cup of chocolate syrup, 2–3 drops of almond extract, and a touch more of rose water. 🌱

RECYCLE!

Being a great recycler and hating to waste all those lovely herbs, I've often tinctured the herbs again, and sometimes even a third time, depending on the strength of the herbs. I have found that I can get a good-quality second tincture, but by the third round, it's pretty weak.

One A Day Male Tonic

This is my version of "one a day," that is, one tablespoon a day. I love to use herbs in food and cooking, rather than always taking them in a medicinal preparation such as tinctures or capsules. Herbal pastes can be spread on toast, licked from the spoon, or added to boiling water for instant tea. Stored in the refrigerator, the paste will last indefinitely. Here's one version of the recipe.

1 part ashwangandha powder

2 parts fo-ti powder

1 part Siberian ginseng powder

1 part astragalus powder

½ part echinacea powder

1 part licorice root powder

¼ part ginger powder

1 part cinnamon powder

1 part cardamom powder

honey

fruit concentrate

Mix all the herbs together in a bowl. Add enough honey and fruit concentrate (blended according to your tastes) to form a paste. Pure rose water also can be added for an exotic flavor. Be sure that the paste is moist enough. It will dry out a bit in the refrigerator, even when tightly closed. If it becomes too dry, moisten with a little more fruit concentrate and honey.

HAVING FUN WITH BASIC RECIPES

One year I wanted to make something special for several of my older neighbors who were going on a holiday cruise. In the midst of making my Energy Balls, some devious little creature took over and they became Aphrodite's Super Aphrodisiac Balls. I added passion-promoting flavors like black cherry liqueur, then a host of aphrodisiac herbs, plus a tablespoon or two of guarana just to keep things moving. The final touch was coating them each in organic bittersweet dipping chocolate. To this day I will walk down the streets of my little Vermont town and strangers will come up to me asking, "Are you the woman who made those balls?" This is always followed by, "Will you make some for me?"

Ginseng Honey with Spice

I often preserve my herbs in the honey pot. Ginseng is especially nice prepared this way. The honey will take on the qualities of the ginseng and can be used in tea and in cooking. Of course, you can mix other herbs in with your ginseng honey. Try fo-ti, astragalus, ashwangandha, and any combination of spices such as ginger, cinnamon, and cardamom, an especially favorite blend of mine.

Occasionally, when using fresh roots, my honey ferments. This will happen if there is a lot of moisture content in the ginseng roots. So, I end up with ginseng honey mead! If you don't want mead (it's rather strong tasting), partially dry your roots before using them.

> fresh ginseng roots
> honey

Slice ginseng roots into rounds and place them in a wide-mouthed jar. Pour warmed honey over them, cover tightly, and let sit for 2–3 weeks.

Herbal Bathing

There are many herbs that can be used in the bath. Get a big bathtub — one of those deep, old claw foots or even a modern Jacuzzi-style one will do — and fill it with water, herbs, and essential oils. Light incense and candles. Serve up that Damiana Chocolate Love Liqueur that you made weeks ago, along with some chocolate-covered strawberries. And in Diana style, sprinkle a path of fresh rose petals leading to the tub that your heart's desire can't refuse to follow. Your heart will be nourished — and perhaps other parts of your body as well.

Deep Relaxation

Try this bath whenever you need to unwind. The recipe makes enough for four to six baths.

    2 parts sage
    2 parts chamomile
    1 part lavender
    1 part hops
    6–8 drops clary sage or lavender essential oil

Mix herbs. Add essential oil and mix well. Place a handful of the mixture in a cotton bag, nylon sock, or strainer and tie on to the nozzle of the tub. Let the hot water run through it for a few minutes. Then release the container into the tub and adjust the temperature of the water. Alternatively, you can prepare a strong herbal tea and add the tea water, after being strained, to the bathwater.

Refreshing/Stimulating Blend

If you need to energize, use this invigorating blend.

    2 parts peppermint
    2 parts rosemary
    6–8 drops pine essential oil

Mix herbs. Add essential oil and mix well. Place a handful of the mixture in a cotton bag, nylon sock, or strainer and tie on to the nozzle of the tub. Let the hot water run through it for a few minutes. Then release the container into the tub and adjust the temperature of the water. Alternatively, you can prepare a strong herbal tea and add the tea water, after being strained, to the bathwater.

Bath Blend for Sore Muscles

Sore muscles will benefit from soaking in this eucalyptus, sage, and pine blend. The recipe makes enough for two to four baths.

- 2 parts eucalyptus leaf
- 2 parts sage
- 6–8 drops pine or sage essential oil

Mix herbs. Add essential oil and mix well. Place a handful of the mixture in a cotton bag, nylon sock, or strainer and tie on to the nozzle of the tub. Let the hot water run through it for a few minutes. Then release the container into the tub and adjust the temperature of the water. Alternatively, you can prepare a strong herbal tea and add the tea water, after being strained, to the bathwater.

ESSENTIAL OILS AND THE BATH

Pure essential oils can enhance the bathing experience enormously. However, be extremely cautious when adding it to the bathwater. I hate to admit it, but my first marriage ended because of a peppermint oil bath! My dear (ex) husband, very ill and feverish, stepped into a therapeutic bath to which I had inadvertently added peppermint instead of eucalyptus oil. The poor innocent let out a squeal that I remember to this day. I always like to remind him that he was, after all, well the next day, but he insists he just never again dared to let me know when he was not feeling well.

chapter six

Remedies for Specific Ailments

In this section we'll cover many of the common health problems men experience and their corresponding natural treatments. Often illness responds simply to rest, a healthy diet, and effective but noninvasive remedies. When a problem doesn't respond to your best efforts, seek the guidance of a health care professional, ideally one knowledgeable and supportive of natural therapies. Remember, the body has its own innate wisdom; learning to listen to and trust our "body knowing" is part of the process of self healing.

Prostatitis and Enlarged Prostate Gland

The prostate is getting a lot of press these days. It may even be the most talked about male organ; it's certainly in the running for second place. Even so, many men are still not sure what it does, or even where it's located unless it starts aching.

A chestnut-shaped organ, no larger than a walnut, the prostate is a part-muscular, part-glandular organ that is located below the bladder and next to the rectum. It surrounds the urethra, the tube that runs from the bladder to the tip of the penis, thus it affects and is affected by the urinary system. If the prostate gets inflamed or engorged and pinches off this tube, bladder infections, urinary incontinence, and kidney problems ensue. The prostate is also directly related to fertility, as it produces and secretes a mysterious protein-like fluid into the semen that is critical for sperm motility.

How to Determine If You Have Prostate Problems

This inconspicuous little organ can cause a lot of problems for men. Nearly 60 percent of the male population between 40 and 60 years old suffers from benign prostatic hyperplasia (BPH), a condition that occurs when the prostate becomes enlarged or engorged. The symptoms of prostatitis (inflammation of the prostate) and BPH are similar:

- Painful urination
- Difficulty in emptying the bladder completely
- Possible blood in the urine
- Reduced force when urinating
- Pain upon sitting
- Unexplained chills and fever

The causes of prostate problems are varied but most are directly related to stress or the man's susceptibility to stress. Oftentimes, though not always, the stress may be of a sexual nature. Irregular sexual patterns can also be a precursor for prostatitis; that is intense sexual activity after a long period of inactivity or a period of inactivity after intense sexual play. It seems the prostate likes regularity. An unhealthy diet, consumption of alcohol and caffeine-rich products, lack of physical exercise, too much sitting, and infections of gums and tonsils, or venereal disease can contribute to prostatitis.

The prostate gland responds incredibly well to home treatments. However, if it doesn't respond within a few days, you'll want to consult a holistic health practitioner or physician. Be aware that you'll need to make several changes in order to treat this ailment.

Dietary Treatments

Eat simple, nourishing foods to enhance prostate health, as well as overall health. Diet should consist primarily of simple steamed vegetables, grains, and miso or chicken soup. Add medicinal herbs such as echinacea, astragalus, fo-ti, and ginseng to the soup base. I usually don't remove the herbs, but just scoop around them.

Include lemon juice and unsweetened cranberry juice in your daily diet. Don't eat foods that you know will further irritate the prostate gland. Caffeine-rich foods, alcohol, and sugar seem to be particularly irritating.

Several foods, vitamins, and minerals are excellent in helping to alleviate prostate enlargement and inflammation.

Include in the diet the following foods:
- Pumpkin seeds (¼ to ½ cup or more daily)
- Cucumbers (2 to 3 daily)
- Calcium/Magnesium (600 mg combined daily)
- Vitamin E (400 I.U. daily)
- Zinc (20 to 50 mg daily)

Watermelon Cooling Tonic

Watermelon seeds are a wonderful remedy for any type of prostate imbalance. If watermelon is in season, you're in luck. Put as much watermelon and seeds as you can drink in one serving in a blender (cut off the rind). Add a handful of unsalted pumpkin seeds. Blend until creamy. Drink a quart daily. Fresh watermelon is wonderful for the kidneys and prostate, providing a mineral-rich flush. If there is a lot of congestion in the gland, this is an excellent cooling tonic.

If watermelon is not in season, you can still make this remedy by using the seeds of the watermelon. Watermelon seeds can be purchased at some herb stores, but why not collect and dry your own in the warm summer months? Place the watermelon seeds and pumpkin seeds in the blender with unsweetened cranberry juice. Blend until creamy. Drink three to four cups daily.

Medicinal Teas

The following two medicinal formulas are excellent remedies for swollen, inflamed prostate. Drink three to four cups daily of one or both formulas. You can also combine 10 drops of saw palmetto tincture with 10 drops of pygeum tincture, dilute in the tea or with warm water, and take three times daily.

Formula One for Prostate Health

1 part uva ursi
1 part cleavers
2 parts nettle
3 parts corn silk
3 parts watermelon seeds

Prepare herbs in an infusion as instructed on page 18.

Formula Two for Prostate Health

- 1 part gravel root
- 1 part saw palmetto (can add a few drops of tincture)
- 1 part echinacea
- 1 part pygeum
- 2 parts marsh mallow root

Prepare herbs in a decoction as instructed on page 19.

Making an Herbal Poultice

Though messy, poultices are very helpful for relieving congestion. Mix equal amounts of clay, comfrey leaf, and slippery elm powder in a bowl with warm water. Place the mixture on a gauze or muslin fabric and apply directly to skin covering the gland twice a day for 20 minutes. Use a jockstrap or underwear to hold the poultice in place.

You can also mix fresh comfrey leaves in a blender with a little water to make a paste, place the mixture on gauze or muslin fabric, and use this as a poultice. If nothing else is available, try an oatmeal poultice.

Hot and Cold Compresses

Hot and cold compresses are also very effective for relieving congestion of the prostate. This treatment requires a bit of willpower. Wrap an ice pack in a towel and place directly on the skin covering the prostate. Leave on for a minute or two. Remove the cold pack and place a hot compress on for a few minutes. Repeat this process three to four times at least once a day.

Another variation of this is a sitz bath, alternating between hot and cold tubs. Drs. Michael T. Murray and Joseph E. Pizzorno, in their excellent book *Encyclopedia of Natural Medicine,* recommend these "contrast baths," stating they're the most beneficial of baths for prostatitis and BPH, but the most difficult to employ. They are very effective for increasing circulation to and improving muscle tone of the prostate and other reproductive organs.

Malignant Prostatic Enlargement (Prostate Cancer)

Until recently, the only accepted treatment for prostate cancer was surgical removal and/or chemotherapy and radiation. Many men who underwent the procedure considered the side effects worse than the cancer. Incontinence, impotence, and depression are just a few of the many possible side effects. Recently, however, conventional medicine has changed its tune about its procedure for prostate cancer and often will recommend a "management program."

Most cancers of the prostate are very slow growing. They can be managed, often slowed down even further, and sometimes go into complete remission. It's easy to monitor prostate enlargement and to know if the cancer is increasing or decreasing in size.

Follow the suggestions listed on the preceding pages for BPH and prostatitis. In addition, add the herbs, foods, and supplements that are known to have cancer-inhibiting properties:

Pau d'Arco is an herb native to South America that has excellent anticarcinogenic properties. It can be taken as capsules, tincture, or tea. I generally blend it in tea, as it has a robust, tasty flavor.

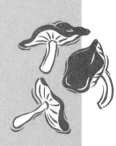

Shiitake and reishi mushrooms both have demonstrated antitumor activity. Though they can be obtained as tinctures and are often found combined in anticancer formulas, shiitake mushrooms are delicious and should be incorporated in one's diet. You can grow them on mushroom logs in your basement, join a shiitake mushroom club and get them delivered to your door, or buy them at most grocery and natural foods stores. Shiitake mushrooms also lower blood cholesterol significantly.

Essiac is a somewhat notorious herbal formula that was known as an old Indian cancer cure. A dedicated nurse, Renee Caisse (Essiac spelled backward) was given the formula to treat cancer patients. She had great success up until the Canadian government forced her to stop using the formula. It went underground for several years and has now surfaced, at outrageous prices, in a flurry of marketing madness. Though not, as marketed, a "cancer cure," it has been known to reduce the size of tumors. It is also highly effective in lessening the painful side effects of conventional cancer therapies. The best sources for high-quality Essiac at reasonable prices are Jean's Greens and Healing Spirits (see Resources).

Glandular and Hormonal Imbalances, Low-Energy, and Lack of Vitality

Lack of energy, depression, infertility, impotence, and lack of vitality characterize glandular imbalance. The usual route is to seek stimulants such as caffeine-rich substances to maintain energy, but these will only further exhaust already depleted energy levels. Instead, try some of the following suggestions to create inner chi and vitality.

- Take Long Life Elixir daily (see recipe on page 53).
- Take two Energy Balls daily (see recipe on page 54).
- Snack on pumpkin seeds, ¼ to ½ cup daily.
- Drink three to four cups of Male Toner Tea daily (see recipe on page 55).
- Eat a small piece of ginseng root daily, or take two ginseng capsules three times daily.
- Take a cold shower at least every other day. I'm a great advocate of cold showers and have found them to be wonderfully restorative. Take a quick warm shower and follow with a cold burst from the faucet. Cold water strengthens the overall constitution of the body and creates greater energy levels. It also stimulates immune function by improving circulation and regulating body temperature.

Impotence and Infertility

Infertility is the inability to conceive after a period of adequate effort (a one-year period, by clinical standards). The latest statistics show that men's systems are the root of at least 40 percent of couples' infertility problems. Most cases of male infertility are due to low sperm count and/or weak or inactive sperm. Stress and lack of activity can be contributing factors. Some less common causes are obstructions in the reproductive system, liver problems, and glandular imbalances in the thyroid (hypothyroidism) or pituitary gland.

Impotence, or erectile dysfunction, afflicts more than 30 million men. A comprehensive men's health study performed in Massachusetts reported that 52 percent of men between the ages of 40 and 70 experience some degree of impotence.

The Introduction of Viagra

With the advent of Viagra, the first pharmaceutical drug found to be effective in treating impotence, one of men's best-kept secrets may have been revealed. Introduced in the early spring of 1998, more than a million prescriptions for Viagra were filled by the end of that year. However, there have been many side effects reported, several deaths related to its use, and no studies have been conducted to determine what its long-term effects on the human body are.

Viagra works by causing the muscles surrounding the penis to relax, thereby increasing blood flow into the spongy tissue comprising the shaft of the penis. While Viagra is effective 60 to 90 percent of the time in producing the desired outcome, it does nothing to correct underlying causes of impotence.

Factors like stress, poor eating habits, high or low blood pressure, mental exhaustion, and possible prostate infection are overlooked. Aging is also considered a cause of impotence in men in their middle years and onward, although I believe it's the unhealthy habits we acquire as we age that create many of the problems associated with the elderly years, including impotence. Lack of exercise, sleep and dreaming, mineral-rich foods, and good relationships, plus many stress factors lead to unhealthy physical changes. Men as well as women have the opportunity to continuously recharge their sexual health by creating good living habits.

How Can Impotence and Infertility Be Treated?

I prefer to use herbs, exercise, and diet to help correct the underlying problems and restore balance to the overall system. The *penis erectis* isn't a solo performer, nor does it

function independently of the rest of the body; it is an indic-
tor of overall well-being. When it refuses to respond, listen to
it. Generally its message is that something is awry — and it's
not always about sex.

- Emphasize the following herbs in your formulas:
  Siberian ginseng, muira puama, saw palmetto, astra-
  galus, ashwangandha, nettles, oats, dandelion, sar-
  saparilla, licorice, wild yam, and fo-ti or ho shou wu
- Follow the suggestions listed for prostate health,
  including use of saw palmetto
- Take 400 I.U. of vitamin E daily
- Take zinc supplements daily (30 ml)
- Take 1 teaspoon of bee pollen daily
- Establish a nonstressful but vigorous daily physical
  exercise program
- Eat lots of fresh raw vegetables, high quality protein,
  fresh fruit, and grains. Avoid all processed refined
  foods, alcohol, sugar, and caffeine-rich foods
- Take two Energy Balls (see recipe on page 54), ¼ cup
  of Long Life Elixir (see recipe on page 53), and 1 to 2
  teaspoons of One A Day Male Tonic (see recipe on
  page 59) daily

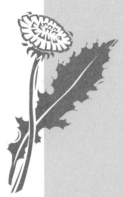

Inflamed Penis or Foreskin Infection

Though inflammation of the foreskin and penis shaft is fairly
uncommon in most circumcised men, I have seen and treated
foreskin infections in babies and young boys. An infected
foreskin can be painfully disruptive.

External Applications

The quickest and most effective action is to make a
powder of three parts slippery elm powder or marsh mallow
root powder to one part organically grown goldenseal powder.
Sprinkle this powder over the head and shaft of the penis.

The Male Herbal author James Green describes how to do
penis soaks, the equivalent of an herbal douche, and thought-
fully instructs on choosing a proper size container. Make a
strong tea of comfrey and organic goldenseal. Pour the warm

tea into a small glass and place the penis in it for as long as possible. (For children, this may be only a few minutes, considering the activity level of most small boys.) As an alternative method, soak a soft cotton cloth in the tea and place it directly on the infected area.

I've also had success clearing up foreskin infections with a wash made of a decoction of witch hazel bark (*not* the extract), white oak bark, and raspberry leaf. Gently wash the infected area two to three times daily with this astringent, disinfectant tea.

Internal Applications

If the infection persists, treat internally with a mixture of organically grown goldenseal or chaparral, echinacea, marsh mallow root, and myrrh. These herbs can be powdered, encapsulated (in size 0 caps), and taken at regular intervals throughout the day (one capsule, three times daily for small children. For infants, mix a pinch of the powder with warm milk or juice. Adults may take two capsules three times daily).

This mixture, useful for many types of infections, can also be tinctured. For a small child or infant, mix three to ten drops of the tincture in warm water, milk, or tea and administer three times daily. For adults, take ¼ teaspoon of the tincture three to six times daily.

Urinary Tract Infections

Weak bladders and urinary tract infections often plague men, most probably due to the placement of that male organ, the prostate. Follow the advice for prostatitis and enlarged prostate glands on pages 64–67. In addition, try the suggestions listed here.

Drink Cranberry Juice

Drink two to four glasses of cranberry juice daily. Cranberries are the natural treatment of choice for the bladder and kidney since they contain a chemical that prevents bacteria from adhering to the urethra wall, thus helping to prevent urinary tract infection.

If you're prone to bladder infections, keep on hand unsweetened cranberry juice. Dilute the tart juice with apple juice or tea. You also can use fresh or frozen cranberries and cranberry tablets for urinary tract infections.

Use Herbs to Support the System

There are a host of wonderful herbs used to support urinary health. For urinary tract infections, include uva ursi, Oregon grape root, and buchu in your herbal formulas. Goldenseal can be effective, but use only organically grown "seal." Couch grass, corn silk, and dandelion leaves are also effective for urinary tract imbalances. Saw palmetto should be included, as it has such a direct and positive impact on the prostate. To soothe inflammation in the urethra, marsh mallow root is the herb of choice. It is an important ingredient in many formulas for bladder or kidney inflammation and infections.

The Importance of Kegels

Kegel exercises are the best strengthening tool we have for toning and conditioning the bladder and entire genitourinary tract. (See page 11 for instructions.) They were designed by a doctor to treat urinary incontinence. If you're prone to bladder infections, the caliber and force of your urine is steadily getting weaker, and you are beginning to "dribble," get on with those kegels immediately.

Yeast Infections

Men, if your partner has a vaginal infection of any kind, chances are you have it too. The problem is that men are often asymptomatic, and partners unwittingly pass the infection back and forth. Women's reproductive organs are like warm petri dishes; living organisms thrive in the warm, deep, moist recesses of the vaginal cave. Yeast and other bacteria tend to grow more quickly and produce more intense symptoms in women than in men with the same infection. No matter how careful a woman is and how committed she is to following a treatment program, it will be futile unless you follow through too.

What to Do

Traditional allopathic medicine isn't always necessary in treating yeast-related infections, and, in fact, will often make the condition worse. Follow these simple guidelines to prevent and treat your yeast infections:

Penis soaks should be done both before and after lovemaking. These are the equivalent to vaginal douches. Follow the instructions on page 71. Enjoy the experience; it's not often that one gets an excuse to hang out in a cup of tea.

Cut back on sugar consumption, since all yeast and yeast-related infections thrive on a sugar-rich diet. Sugars — whether from candy bars, white cane sugar, raisins, dates, mangoes, oranges, or a chocolate-covered granola bar — create an acidic condition and a perfect medium for bacteria to grow in.

Eat an alkalizing diet consisting of dark green leafy vegetables, miso, fish, organically raised chicken, soy protein, seitan, salads, root vegetables, and cultured milk products such as yogurt, buttermilk, and kefir.

Use herbs that build immunity such as echinacea and astragalus, herbs that fight infection such as organically grown goldenseal or chaparral, and herbs that soothe irritated reproductive tissue such as marsh mallow root. These herbs can be powdered and taken daily in capsules, made into tinctures, or served as tea.

Minimize your dairy intake. Dairy products (except for cultured milk products) such as milk and cheeses are also acidic and will promote infection.

Inguinal Hernia

Though not normally classified as a male health problem, far more men than women get hernias. This could be because of heavy lifting or straining or because the tissue or muscle at the lower end of the abdominal cavity is either congenitally weak or becomes weak and loosens, leaving an opening through which a loop of the intestines protrudes. Inguinal hernias are most often noticed as a lump protruding from the lower abdomen and sometimes a pain that radiates from the groin. The pain can get quite severe. Chronic constipation can also exacerbate inguinal hernias, since the straining will create extra pressure.

To Treat Hernias

Apply clay packs twice daily over the hernia. Any clay will do, but my preference for medicinal purposes is green volcanic clay. Mix the clay into a paste with water and apply directly to the hernia. Cover with a cotton cloth and hold in place with an ace bandage. Hernia supports can be obtained at most medical supply stores. The clay poultice can be wrapped in gauze and placed inside the support belt. Wear this for at least an hour a day, longer if it's not too uncomfortable.

Take 2,000 mg of vitamin C daily. Drink herb teas that are astringent and healing. The following tea is recommended in doses of three to four cups daily:

Oatstraw and Horsetail Remedy

1 part oatstraw	2 parts lemon balm
1 part horsetail	2 parts white oak bark
2 parts nettle	4 parts comfrey leaf
3 parts raspberry	(optional)

Make an infusion of the herbs by following the directions on page 18. 🌸

COMFREY CONTROVERSY

There is a current, as yet unresolved controversy surrounding the use of comfrey for internal purposes. Generally, I no longer recommend comfrey internally for others, though I continue to use it myself abundantly. In the case of hernias, because of its extreme usefulness in healing torn or damaged tissue, I am braving the wrath of the herbal community and including it in the formula. Please educate yourself as to the controversy, and make up your own mind. For further information you can send a SASE to my address or write to the Herb Research Foundation (see Resources).

Avoid all lifting and straining, and do not allow constipation to be a contributing factor to your hernia. Drink plenty of water and gentle herbal bowel tonics such as psyllium, yellow dock root, and licorice root. Use small amounts of senna or cascara sagrada blended with fennel and licorice root for serious constipation.

Heart Problems

In order to stop breaking our hearts we will have to start breaking our male rules.

— T.E.S.

I find it so sad that the heart, that great throbbing center of emotions and feelings, is the number one killer of men today. I know that this is in part because of "heart unfriendly" dietary patterns established in this century and because most men no longer work as hard physically or get the exercise they did a hundred years ago. We know that stress levels are up as we near the end of a millennium and contemplate enormous changes on this planet that will affect life for centuries hereafter. That's a lot of weight on a man's heart.

But the real reason for this rash of heart disease and troubled hearts may be less obvious, or less talked about. In the novel *The English Patient,* there was a poignant line that struck me: "The heart is an organ of fire." The heart is fed and nourished by love, touch, and feeling, sensory experiences that many men are lacking. Love, touch, bonding, feelings so enormously important to the human heart are often lacking or completely devoid in the workplace of most men. Oftentimes, home doesn't provide that intimate heart energy either.

Sadly, most men don't even recognize this as a problem. But heart disease continues to rise. Dr. Dean Ornish, in his outstanding book *Dr. Dean Ornish's Program for Reversing Heart Disease,* offers excellent counsel on heart disease. His advice goes far beyond dietary and exercise measures and explores the realms of "maleness" in our society and its effect on heart disease. Sam Keene and Robert Bly are other authors whose insights into men's hearts are worth exploring.

Maintaining Heart Health

It is quite amazing what effects herbs, good dietary measures, and plenty of the right kind of nourishment (i.e., lots of love, caring, and touching) can have on men with heart conditions.

Herbs for Heart Disease

Hawthorn, in its many delicious forms, is an absolute must. Include it as a food, tea, and medicine (tinctures and capsules) daily. Studies in Europe have verified its ability to reduce angina attacks as well as lowering blood pressure and serum cholesterol levels. Hawthorn is a food herb and can be used safely with heart medication.

Other tonic herbs that are specific for heart health are motherwort, garlic, valerian, cayenne, and yarrow. Each of these herbs has a specific toning effect on the heart. Use your herbal reference guides to explore each of these herbs in more detail. When on heart medication be very cautious about which herbs and supplements you use. Though this list comprises benevolent and safe herbs, it is wise when working with heart problems to work in conjunction with a holistic health care practitioner, who can provide insights on the best formulas for your particular constitution and condition.

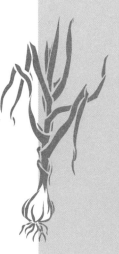

Dietary Factors and Supplements

Diet is critical to the health of the heart. There are so many good publications and books about the effects of diet on the heart that I'll only remind you of its importance here and steer you toward the works of Dr. Dean Ornish and others. Evaluate your diet thoroughly and throw out those things you know are destroying your heart. While you're at it, you might evaluate the rest of your life and begin to clear out or change whatever else may be causing you pain and heartache.

Supplement with 20 to 30 mg of coenzyme Q10. This natural substance found in most foods assists in oxidative metabolism and seems to improve the utilization of oxygen at a cellular level. People with poor circulation and heart problems seem to benefit most from it.

"MEDICINE" FOR THE HEART

While visiting with my longtime friend and farmer extraordinaire, Tim Blakley, we were reminiscing about the "good old days at herb school," which ultimately led to dreaming about future plans. I've known Tim since he was in his early 20s; he's now in his mid-40s. He still looks 20, really. He's trim and fit with a radiant sparkle in his eyes. His dreams for the near future? To spend a summer hiking the Pacific Crest Trail with his wife, Heather. And they're already planning it. It's a good way to stay fit and trim, as well as the best way to commune with nature. Good heart medicine all the way around.

Exercise!

One of the most important factors in building and maintaining a healthy heart is exercise. James Green states that "exercise alone may be the most effective non-drug method for normalizing blood pressure." Lack of exercise and a diet high in rich, fatty foods that packs on extra poundage (take a look at the "normal" American male's diet) is a deadly combination.

Take your heart out for a walk today. Keep lean and trim as you grow older if your heart is at stake. Exercise comes in many forms, from simple stretches to vigorous workouts at the gym, to yoga and sports. All are good. Never forget the importance of life exercise where you exchange energy with the natural world as you're hiking, biking, running, or stretching fully in response to your own body's need to move.

Hypertension

A disease of modern civilization, hypertension, or high blood pressure, is one of the major medical problems of the twentieth century. It is directly related to cardiovascular disease, angina, and heart attacks. Although 92 percent of all diagnosed hypertension is termed essential (i.e., the underlying mechanism is unknown), the primary cause is almost always directly related to diet, stress, and lifestyle choices, with diet being the primary factor. Hypertension is almost unknown in undeveloped regions of the world where people still enjoy a diet untainted by fast food and other culinary wonders of modern civilization. In these areas hypertension is not an accepted aspect of aging, as it is in more developed countries.

Treating Hypertension Naturally

Unnecessary body weight, caffeine, alcohol, stresses, smoking, and lack of exercise are major factors contributing to hypertension in individuals. Given the wide range of side effects attributed to antihypertensive medication — including impotence and exhaustion — it seems well worthwhile to consider lifestyle changes related to the above factors. According to long-term clinical studies reported by the American Medical Association and the *American Journal of Cardiology,* people taking blood pressure medication actually fared worse than those with hypertension who didn't take medication.

For dietary suggestions and lifestyle modifications for hypertension, consult *Dr. Dean Ornish's Program for Reversing Heart Disease.*

When treating hypertension consider the following:

Garlic is among the most effective herbs for normalizing blood pressure levels. Eat it raw, chopped, and added to salad dressings. Odorless encapsulated garlic works well also. Other helpful herbs are motherwort, vervain, yarrow, shiitake mushrooms, Siberian ginseng, onions, and hawthorn.

Coenzyme Q10 plays a significant role in metabolic processes involved with energy production. Individuals with cardiovascular disease and hypertension show decreased levels of coenzyme Q10. Supplements are available.

Essential fatty acids, especially those found in black currant seeds, flaxseed, and evening primrose have a profound effect on hypertension. Flaxseed can be ground and added to food. (Store in the refrigerator to reduce rancidity.)

Mistletoe is one of the most widely used herbs for hypertension in Europe, where it is frequently combined with hawthorn. However, mistletoe can be very toxic, even in moderate doses. Use only under the supervision of a competent herbalist or naturopathic doctor.

High-potassium herbs such as dandelion leaf have a mild diuretic action and work as a kidney tonic as well. The health of the heart is directly connected to the health of the kidneys.

Herpes

Herpes is not a gender specific "evil"; it seems to thrive in both sexes. Unfortunately, this nasty little virus is prevalent everywhere in our society. Few people have not experienced it in some form or another either as cold sores, shingles, or herpes simplex I or II. I've seen terrible cases covering the bottoms of little children and a painful outbreak hiding the entire face of a beautiful woman.

The Best Remedy: Licorice Root

Licorice root extract or tincture has been my most successful remedy for clearing up herpes simplex I and II. Licorice inhibits both the growth and the cell-damaging effects of herpes. Amanda McQuade Crawford, incredible herbalist and friend, shared this remedy with me several years ago and I have recommended it many times since to others. It's best applied several times a day with a cotton ball or swab *immediately* upon the first signs of the outbreak. When I used it on my fever blister, the sore was completely gone in two days.

Other Treatments

If you learn to pay attention to your body and the unique signals "your herpes" sends out, you can often prevent an outbreak from happening. Herpes doesn't just occur. It is highly unusual for there not to be a series of "smoke alarms" or signals that the body sends out loud and clear if we're willing to pay attention.

Immediately, upon the first signals of a herpes outbreak, follow these guidelines:
- Stop eating any sweets and foods high in the amino acid arginine such as peanuts, peanut butter, chocolate, coffee, coconut, grains, and carob. If

not actually the cause, these foods will most surely agitate a herpes outbreak. At the same time increase lysine-rich foods such as nutritional yeast, eggs, milk, and beans. Many people feel it beneficial to take lysine supplements: three 500-milligram tablets three times a day during the outbreak. Do not continue on this high-dose lysine program for longer than a few days.

- Begin taking high doses of echinacea tincture: ¼ teaspoon of the tincture every hour throughout the day.
- Apply an ice pack directly to the lesion. Repeat several times during the day until all symptoms subside.
- Apply licorice root extract or tincture to the area. Other herbs that have good reputations as antiviral medications for herpes are lemon balm (especially the essential oil), tea tree oil, bergamot oil (which can cause photosensitivity, so be careful), and St.-John's-wort oil (helpful for reducing the pain of herpes). A good remedy combines the tinctures of St.-John's-wort, licorice extract, and calendula. Mix in equal amounts and apply frequently throughout the day. The tincture combination should also be taken internally; use ½ to 1 teaspoon 3 times a day. If using the remedy externally, apply several times daily with a cotton ball or swab.
- Apply Kloss's goldenseal liniment. This is an old, very strong recipe combining equal parts of organically cultivated goldenseal, myrrh, and echinacea with ¼ part cayenne (all in powder form). Place powders in a jar and cover with rubbing alcohol (a food-grade alcohol can be used, but rubbing alcohol seems to work best), leaving a good two-inch margin above the herbs. Put a tight-fitting lid on and let the mixture sit in a warm place for four weeks. Strain, rebottle, and label. If you've used rubbing alcohol, be sure to write in large, bold letters EXTERNAL USE ONLY. Dilute with a little water if you experience a stinging sensation upon application.

    You've just made one of the finest disinfectant remedies you'll ever have on hand. For herpes, you might wish to add essential oil of lemon balm and extract of licorice root for added antiviral activities. This disinfectant also can be used as an external wound cleanser, for swellings and infections, and for insect bites.

- Drink nervine herbs throughout the herpes outbreak: passionflower, skullcap, chamomile, lemon balm, and lavender. Be kind to yourself. Usually a herpes outbreak is a signal that you're "stressing," so lighten your load, don't add to it.

Depression and Anxiety

Depression and anxiety certainly aren't unique to men, and even though, statistically, more women are clinically depressed than men, when men fall in the grips of depression, they fall hard. Perhaps it's because I'm middle-aged now (just turned 50!), and many of my friends, men and women, are also in this transitory stage of life, that I've noticed more men going through major stages of depression. Though anxiety and depression are technically different, I see them as symptoms of the same imbalance and use similar treatment protocols for both.

Depression is marked by varying degrees of either insomnia or hypersomnia, appetite irregularities (either excessive weight gain or loss), loss of energy accompanied by a sense of fatigue, diminished ability to think clearly, and general loss of interest in life. Though there are many and complex reasons for depression, herbs and nutrition can help all types of depression. In fact, along with supportive counseling, nutritional support with a strong emphasis on biogenic amines (also known as monoamines) is becoming one of the most effective ways to treat depression.

The biogenic amine hypothesis links biochemical derangements such as depression with imbalances of amino acids in the delicate ecology of our system. Amino acids are essential to the healthy formation of neurotransmitters, complex compounds that form communication links between the nerve cells. Many practitioners are including biogenic amines with other holistic therapies to successfully treat depression. Results are promising. For a more in-depth discussion of biogenic amine therapy for the treatment of depression, see the *Encyclopedia of Natural Medicine* by Drs. Michael T. Murray and Joseph E. Pizzorno.

St.-John's-wort Remedy

Probably the most promising herb for depression is St.-John's-wort. Though marketed as if it's a recent discovery, St.-John's-wort has been used for centuries for depression, anxiety, and nerve damage. It's interesting that the American public woke up and discovered St.-John's-wort at the same time that Prozac and Zoloft are being consumed like candy. At least it offers an effective alternative for those choosing to manage their nervous stress differently.

St.-John's-wort works best for mild depression, though it can be used for clinical cases as part of an overall program supported by diet, counseling, and exercise. For depression, take ½ teaspoon of St.-John's-wort three to four times daily or, if in capsules, two caps three times daily. Many people recommend extracts standardized to 0.3 percent hypericin, but I have found the whole plant extract works as well when prepared properly. St.-John's-wort definitely has that ability to brighten one's day. It should be used for three to four weeks before deciding if it does or doesn't work for you.

Other Important Herbal Therapies

St.-John's-wort has gained such fame as an antidepressant that it has eclipsed other important nervine herbs. Oats (leafy tops, stalks, and oatmeal) are an incredible herb for depression and anxiety. They slowly and surely build the myelin sheath of the nerves, reducing stress and irritability. Passionflower is another herb indicated for nerve stress that strengthens and tones the entire nervous system. Combine it with oats, lemon balm, and St.-John's-wort for an excellent antidepressant tea. Valerian can help regulate sleep, while ginseng, astragalus, licorice, and ashwangandha help energize the system on a cellular level.

Implement an Overall Health Care Program

Depression, though often associated with loss and emotions, may be more closely related to chemical imbalances in our body that are helped by herbs, supplements, rest, diet, and exercise. The proper diet makes a big difference; during times of depression and anxiety, find a holistic health care practitioner who can help you create a nutritional supplement program to support you through the critical stages of the illness.

Exercise is an important component of any program for depression. Find a routine that you can stick to. Though gym-type exercise is fine, nothing lifts the spirits more than interacting with nature: walking, hiking, bike riding, canoeing. Take your cares to Mother Earth and the great healing spirit of nature.

LISTEN TO YOURSELF

I also suspect that depression may be an indicator or wake-up call, a sign that we're alive and well and at least attempting to respond sanely to an insane situation. I've found that the times I've been most depressed have been when I was not listening to some deep biological song within me, that place that holds the dream sacred, and follows no matter what. A more manly way to explain this might be to say that when you know you've got to do something, stop resisting and just do it. Follow your heart; it is the pathway to the soul.

Recommended Reading

It must be noted that among the ever-growing number of herb books on women's health, there are only two available on men's health. It's such a pity. I am including a number of other excellent herb books that will shed some light on the subject.

Buhner, Stephen. *Sacred Plant Medicine.* Boulder, CO: Roberts Rhinehart Publishers, 1996.

Cowen, Eliot. *Plant Spirit Medicine.* Newberg, OR: Swan, Raven & Company, 1995.

DeLuca, Diana. *Botanica Erotica: Arousing Body, Mind & Spirit.* Rochester, VT: Healing Arts Press, 1998.

Fallon, Sally. *Nourishing Traditions.* San Diego, CA: ProMotion Publishing, 1995.

Green, James. *The Male Herbal.* Freedom, CA: The Crossing Press, 1991.

Hobbs, Christopher. *Foundations of Health.* Capitola, CA: Botanica Press, 1992.

———. *The Ginsengs.* Santa Cruz, CA: Botanica Press, 1996.

———. *Stress and Natural Healing.* Loveland, CO: Interweave Press, 1997.

Keville, Kathi. *Herbs: An Illustrated Encyclopedia.* New York, NY: Michael Friedman/Fairfax Publishing, 1994.

Mowry, Daniel. *Herbal Tonic Therapies.* New Canaan, CT: Keats Publishing, 1993.

Murray, Michael T., and Joseph E. Pizzorno, N.D. *Encyclopedia of Natural Medicine.* Rockland, CA: Prima Publishing, 1991.

Pedersen, Mark. *Nutritional Herbology.* Warsaw, IN: Wendell Whitman Co., 1994.

Pitchford, Paul. *Healing with Whole Foods.* Berkeley, CA: North Atlantic Books, 1993.

Teeguarden, Ron. *Chinese Tonic Herbs.* New York: Japan Publications, 1984.

Wood, Matthew. *The Book of Herbal Wisdom.* Berkeley, CA: North Atlantic Books, 1998.

Resources

Where to Find Herbs

Thankfully, herbs and herbal products are now widely available. I generally suggest purchasing herbal products from local sources, as it helps support bioregional herbalism and community-based herbalists. However, here are some of my favorite sources for high-quaility herbs and herbal products.

Frontier Herbs

P.O. Box 299
Norway, IA 52318
(800) 669-3275
Aside from having an incredible list of supplies and herbs, Frontier emphasizes medicinal plant conservation and preservation. Frontier is a wholesale supplier, but offers price breaks for individual buyers.

Green Mountain Herbs

P.O. Box 532
Putney, VT 05436
(888) 4GRNMTS

Healing Spirits

9198 State Route 415
Avoca, NY 14809
(607) 566-2701
One of the best sources of ethically wildcrafted and organically grown herbs in the northeast.

Jean's Greens

119 Sulphur Springs Road
Newport, NY 13146
(315) 845-6500
A wonderful selection of fresh and dried organic and wild-crafted herbs. Also, oils, containers, beeswax, and other materials needed for making herbal products.

Mountain Rose

20818 High Street
North San Juan, CA 95960
(800) 879-3337
A small herb company nestled in the coastal mountains of northern California, that supplies bulk herbs, beeswax, books, oils, and containers.

Trinity Herbs

P.O. Box 1001
Graton, CA 95444
(707) 824-2040
Trinity is a small wholesale herb company that sells bulk herbs in quantities of one pound or more.

Wild Weeds

1302 Camp Weott Road
Ferndale, CA 95536
(800) 553-9453
A small herbal emporium, this mail-order business was initially started to supply correspondence-course students with the herbs and herbal materials they needed.

Woodland Essences
P.O. Box 206
Cold Brook, NY 13324
(315) 845-1515

Handmade Herbal Products

Each of the following companies provides high-quality herbal products. Write for their current catalogs and price lists.

Avena Botanicals
20 Mill Street
Rockland, ME 04841

Equinox Botanicals
33446 McCumber Road
Rutland, OH 45775

Green Terrestrial
P.O. Box 266
Milton, NY 12547

Herb Pharm
Box 116
Williams, OR 97544

Herbalists and Alchemists
P.O. Box 553
Broadway, NJ 08808

Sage Mountain Herb Products
General Delivery
Lake Elmore, VT 05657
(802) 888-7278
Rosemary Gladstar's company.

Simpler's Botanicals
P.O. Box 39
Forestville, CA 95436

Zand Herbal Products
Products available in most natural foods and herb stores.

Educational Resources

A few years ago it was difficult to find herbal educational opportunities, but today the choices are many. Following are a few well-known herbal schools and programs.

American Herb Association (AHA)
P.O. Box 1673
Nevada City, CA 95959
More complete listings of schools, programs, seminars, and correspondence courses offered throughout the United States. There is a small fee for this publication.

American Herbalist Guild (AHG)
Box 746555
Arvada, CO 80006
More complete listings of schools, programs, seminars, and correspondence courses offered throughout the United States. There is a small fee for this publication.

The California School of Herbal Studies
P.O. Box 39
Forestville, CA 95476
One of the oldest and most respected herb schools in the United States, founded by Rosemary Gladstar in 1982.

Herb Research Foundation
1007 Pearl Street, Suite 200
Boulder, CO 80302
An excellent resource and research organization. They also have a newsletter.

**The Northeast Herb
Association**
P.O. Box 10
Newport, NY 13416

**Rocky Mountain Center
for Botanical Studies**
1705 Fourteenth Street, #287
Boulder, CO 80302
*Offers excellent programs
for beginners, as well as
advanced clinical training
programs.*

**Sage Mountain Retreat
Center and Botanical
Sanctuary**
P.O. Box 420
East Barre, VT 05649
*Apprentice programs and
classes with Rosemary
Gladstar and other well-
known herbalists.*

**The Science and Art
of Herbalism: A Home
Study Course**
by Rosemary Gladstar
P.O. Box 420
East Barre, VT 05649
*The Science and Art of
Herbalism was written in an
inspiring and joyful manner
for students wishing a system-
atic, in-depth study of herbs.
The course emphasizes the
foundations of herbalism,
wildcrafting, Earth awareness, and herbal preparation
and formulation. The heart
of the course is the develop-
ment of a deep personal rela-
tionship with the plant world.*

Herb Newsletters

***The American Herb
Association Newsletter***
P.O. Box 1673
Nevada City, CA 95959

Business of Herbs
North Winds Farm
439 Pondersona Way
Jemez Springs, NM 87025

***Foster's Botanical and
Herb Reviews***
P.O. Box 106
Eureka Springs, AR 72632

HerbalGram
P.O. Box 201660
Austin, TX 78720

The Herb Quarterly
P.O. Box 548
Boiling Springs, PA 17007

***Herbs for Health** and
The Herb Companion*
201 East Fourth Street
Loveland, CO 80537

Medical Herbalism
P.O. Box 33080
Portland, OR 97233

***Planetary Formula
Newsletter***
c/o Roy Upton
P.O. Box 533
Soquel, CA 95073

United Plant Savers
P.O. Box 420
East Barre, VT 05649

Wild Foods Forum
4 Carlisle Way NE
Atlanta, GA 30308

United Plant Savers At-Risk List

United Plant Savers (UpS) is a nonprofit, grassroots organization dedicated to preserving native American medicinal plants and the land that they grow on. An organization for herbalists and people who love and use plants, our purpose is to ensure the future of our rich diversity of medicinal plants through organic cultivation, sustainable wildcrafting practices, creating botanical sanctuaries for medicinal plant conservation, and reestablishing native plant communities in their natural environments.

The following herbs have been designated as "UpS At Risk" due to overharvesting, loss of habitat, or by nature of their innate rareness or sensitivity. UpS is not asking for a moratorium on the use of these herbs, but rather is asking for a concerted effort by all those who use plants as medicine to seek sustainable alternatives; that is, grow your own, buy from reputable companies, or substitute other herbs whenever possible.

American Ginseng *(Panax quinquefolius)*
Black Cohosh *(Cimicifuga racemosa)*
Bloodroot *(Sanguinaria canadensis)*
Blue Cohosh *(Caulophyllum thalictroides)*
Echinacea (*Echinacea* species)
Goldenseal *(Hydrastis canadensis)*
Helonias Root *(Chamaelirium luteum)*
Kava Kava *(Piper methysticum)* (Hawaii only)
Lady's-Slipper (*Cypripedium* species)
Lomatium *(Lomatium dissectum)*
Osha (*Ligusticum porteri* and related species)
Partridgeberry *(Mitchella repens)*
Peyote *(Lophophora williamsii)*
Slippery elm *(Ulmus rubra)*
Sundew (*Drosera* species)
Trillium, Beth root (*Trillium* species)
True Unicorn *(Aletris farinosa)*
Venus's-flytrap *(Dionaea muscipula)*
Wild Yam (*Dioscorea villosa* and related species)

For more information on United Plant Savers and how you can become involved in "Planting the Future," contact United Plant Savers, P.O. Box 98, East Barre, VT 05649; (802) 479-9825; E-mail: info@www.plantsavers.org.

Index

Allopathic medicine, 4–5
Anxiety, 82–84
Ashwangandha *(Withania somnifera)*, 27, 52, 55, 59, 71, 83
Astragalus, 55, 59, 65, 71, 74, 83

Baths, 24, 60–62, 67
Bee pollen, 71
Bergamot oil, 81
Buchu, 73

Calendula, 81
Capsules, herbal, 20–21
Cascara sagrada, 14, 76
Cayenne, 77
Chai Hombre, 57
Chamomile, 61, 82
Chaparral, 74
Chaste tree *(Vitex agnus-castus)*, 28
Chickweed, 14
Clay, 75
Cleavers, 14, 66
Coenzyme Q10, 77, 79
Comfrey, 67, 71, 75
Compresses, hot and cold, 67, 81
Constipation, 75, 76
Corn silk, 66, 73
Couch grass, 73
Cranberry juice, 72–73

Damiana Chocolate Love Liqueur, 58
Damiana *(Turnera aphrodisiaca)*, 28–29, 52, 53, 55, 56
Dandelion, 71, 73, 80
Decoctions, 19
Deep Relaxation, 61
Depression, 69, 82–84
Diet, 9, 65–66, 71, 74, 78–79, 80–81
Disinfectant remedies, 81–82
Dosage, 15–16

Echinacea, 59, 65, 67, 72, 74, 81
Eleuthero. *See* Ginseng, Siberian
Energy, low, 69
Energy Balls, 54, 69, 71
Essential fatty acids, 79
Essiac, 68–69
Eucalyptus, 62
Exercise, 8–9, 11, 73, 78

Fertility and Potency Syrup, 52
Foreskin infection, 71–72
Fo-ti, 53, 55, 57, 59, 65, 71

Garlic, 77, 79
Ginger *(Zingiber officinale)*, 29–30, 53, 57
Ginkgo *(Ginkgo biloba)*, 30–31, 54, 56
Ginseng, American *(Panax quinquefolia)*, 31
Ginseng, Asian *(Panax spp.)*, 32, 53
Ginseng, nonspecific, 52, 54, 55, 56, 57, 65, 69, 83
Ginseng, Siberian *(Eleutherococcus senticosus)*, 33, 54, 55, 59, 71, 79
Ginseng Honey with Spice, 60
Ginseng Tonic Tea, 56–57
Glandular imbalances, 69
Goldenseal, 71, 72, 73, 74, 81–82
Gotu kola, 54
Gravel root, 67

Hawthorn *(Crataegus spp.)*, 34–35, 56, 77, 79
Heart disease, 76–78
Herbalism, 6, 26–27
Hernias, inguinal, 74–76
Herpes, 80–82
Hops, 36, 61
Hormonal imbalances, 69
Horsetail, 75
Ho shou wu, 71
Hypertension, 78–80

Impotence, 69–71
Infections, 82
Infertility, 69–71
Infusions, 18–19
Insect bites, 82

Kava-kava *(Piper methysticum)*, 37
Kegel exercises, 11, 73

Lavender, 61, 82
Lemon balm, 56, 75, 81, 82, 83
Licorice *(Glycyrrhiza glabra)*, 38–39, 53, 55, 57, 59, 71, 76, 80, 81, 82, 83

Long Life Elixir, 53, 69, 71
Lysine, 81

Male Toner Tea, 55, 69
Marsh mallow, 67, 73, 74
Measurements, of herbs, 17
Mistletoe, 79
Motherwort, 77, 79
Muira puama (Ptychopetalum ola-
    coides, Liriosma ovata), 39, 52,
    55, 71
Muscles, Bath Blend for Sore, 62
Mushrooms, 68, 79
Myrrh, 72

Nettles (Urtica dioica), 40–41, 52,
    56, 66, 71, 75

Oats (Avena sativa, A. fatua), 41,
    52, 56, 67, 71, 83
Oatstraw and Horsetail Remedy, 75
One A Day Male Tonic, 59, 71
Onions, 79
Oregon grape root, 73
Orrisroot, 14

Passionflower, 82, 83
Pastes, herbal, 59
Pau d'arco, 68
Penis, inflamed, 71–72
Peppermint, 61
Pine, 61, 62
Plants, at-risk, 43
Potassium, 80
Poultices, 67
Powders, herb, 21
Prostate, enlarged, 64–67
Prostate cancer, 47, 68–69
Prostate Health, Formula One for, 66
Prostate Health, Formula Two for, 67
Prostatitis, 64–67
Psyllium, 76
Pumpkin (Cucurbita pepo), 42
Pumpkin seeds, 54, 69
Pygeum (Pygeum africanum),
    42–43, 66, 67

Quality, of herbs, 14–15

Red raspberry (Rubus idaeus), 44,
    52, 56, 72, 75
Refreshing/Stimulating Blend, 61
Rosemary, 61

Sage, 61, 62
Sarsaparilla (Smilax officinalis),
    44–45, 53, 55, 71
Sassafras (Sassafras albidum),
    45–46, 53, 55
Saw palmetto (Serenoa serrulata,
    S. repens), 46–47, 52, 53, 66, 67,
    71, 73
Senna, 76
Sitz baths, 67
Skullcap, 82
Slippery elm, 67, 71, 72
Spirulina, 54
St.-John's-wort, 81, 83
Standardized extracts, 35
Storage, of herbs, 15
Stress, 82
Swelling, 82
Syrups, herbal, 23, 52

Teas, herbal, 18–20. See also spe-
    cific teas, herbs, or illnesses
Tea tree oil, 81
Tinctures, 21–23, 58

Urinary tract infections, 72–73
Uva ursi, 66, 73

Valerian (Valeriana officinalis),
    47–48, 77, 83
Vervain, 79
Viagra, 70
Vital-a-Tea, Male, 56
Vitality, lack of, 69
Vitamin C, 75
Vitamin E, 71

Watermelon seeds, 66
Wellness, 8–11
White oak bark, 72, 75
Wild yam (Dioscorea villosa), 49, 52,
    53, 55, 71
Wine, Good Life, 55
Witch hazel bark, 72

Yang/yin, 12
Yarrow, 77, 79
Yeast infections, 73–74
Yellow dock, 76
Yohimbe (Pausinystalia yohimbe,
    Corynanthe yohimbe), 49–50

Zinc, 71

Other Storey Books
You Will Enjoy

Also in the Rosemary Gladstar Series: *Herbal Remedies for Children's Health,* ISBN 1-58017-153-2; *Herbs for Longevity and Well-Being,* ISBN 1-58017-154-0; *Herbs for Natural Beauty,* ISBN 1-58017-152-4; *Herbs for Reducing Stress and Anxiety,* ISBN 1-58017-155-9; and *Herbs for the Home Medicine Chest,* ISBN 1-58017-156-7.

Healing with Herbs, by Penelope Ody. This visual introduction to the world of herbal medicine offers clear, illustrated instructions for growing, preparing, and administering healing herbs to relieve a variety of ailments. 160 pages. Hardcover. ISBN 1-58017-144-3.

Herbal Antibiotics, by Stephen Harrod Buhner. This book presents all the current information about antibiotic-resistant microbes and the herbs that are most effective in fighting them. Readers will also find detailed, step-by-step instructions for making and using herbal infusions, tinctures, teas, and salves to treat various types of infections. 128 pages. Paperback. ISBN 1-58017-148-6.

The Herbal Home Remedy Book, by Joyce A. Wardwell. Discover how to use 25 common herbs to make simple herbal remedies. Native American legends and folklore are spread throughout the book. 176 pages. Paperback. ISBN 1-58017-016-1.

Herbal Remedy Gardens, by Dorie Byers. An introduction to more than 20 herbs, their medicinal uses, propagation, and harvesting techniques, this book includes dozens of easy-to-make recipes for common ailments. 38 illustrated garden plans offer choices for customizing a garden to fit your special health needs. 224 pages. Paperback. ISBN 1-58017-095-1.

Making Herbal Dream Pillows, by Jim Long. In this lavishly illustrated book, you'll find step-by-step instructions for creating 15 herbal dream blends and pillows for custom-made dreams. Author Jim Long also explores the history of dream pillows and their ties to folk medicine and herbal mythology. 64 pages. Hardcover. ISBN 1-58017-075-7.

Natural First Aid, by Brigitte Mars. This book offers natural first-aid suggestions for everything from ant bites to wounds. Readers will also find recipes for simple home remedies using herbs, vitamins, essential oils, and foods. Includes an herb profile section detailing the healing properties of common herbs. 128 pages. Paperback. ISBN 1-58017-147-8.

These and other Storey books are available at your bookstore, farm store, garden center, or directly from Storey Books, Schoolhouse Road, Pownal, Vermont 05261, or by calling 1-800-441-5700. Or visit our Web site at www.storey.com.